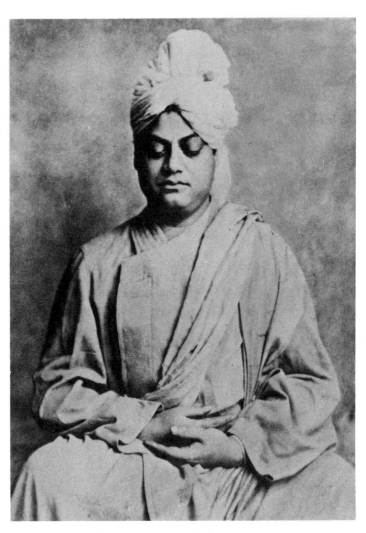

VIVEKANANDA IN MEDITATION

RĀJA-YOGA

by

SWAMI VIVEKANANDA

REVISED EDITION

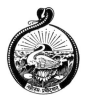

RAMAKRISHNA-VIVEKANANDA CENTER

NEW YORK

RĀJA-YOGA

FIRST EDITION
(Three Printings)

SECOND EDITION
(Four Printings)

PAPERBACK EDITION 1982
(Five Printings)

ISBN 0-911206-23-X

Library of Congress Catalog Card Number: 55-12231

PREFACE

The present revised edition of *Rāja-Yoga* has been taken from *Vivekananda: The Yogas and Other Works,* published in 1953 by the Ramakrishna-Vivekananda Center of New York. The following lines quoted from my preface to the latter will explain the reasons for the editing of the book:

"Swami Vivekananda's public life covered a period of ten years—from 1893, when he appeared at the Parliament of Religions held in Chicago, to 1902, when he gave up his mortal body. These were years of great physical and mental strain as a result of extensive travels, adaptation to new environments, opposition from detractors both in his native land and abroad, incessant public lectures and private instruction, a heavy correspondence, and the organizing of the Ramakrishna Order in India. Hard work and ascetic practices undermined his health. The Swami thus had no time to revise his books, which either were dictated by him or consisted of lectures delivered without notes and taken down in shorthand or longhand. . . . I have therefore felt the need of editing the present collection, making changes wherever they were absolutely necessary, but being always mindful to keep intact the Swami's basic thought."

New material, in the form of two lectures and one article by Swami Vivekananda, has been added in

order to make the present volume uniform with the
other three books of the series.

NIKHILANANDA

Ramakrishna-Vivekananda Center
New York
September 19, 1955

CONTENTS

MISCELLANEOUS

Note on the Pronunciation of Sanskrit and Vernacular Words

a	has the sound of *o* in *come*.
ā	" " " " *a* in *far*.
e	" " " " *e* in *bed*.
i	" " " " *ee* in *feel*.
o	" " " " *o* in *note*.
u	" " " " *u* in *full*.
ai, ay	" " " " *oy* in *boy*.
au	" " " " *o* pronounced deep in the throat.
ch	" " " " *ch* in *church*.
ḍ	" " " " hard *d* (in English).
g	" " " " *g* in *god*.
jn	" " " " hard *gy* (in English).
ś	" " " " *sh* in *shut*.
th	" " " " *t-h* in *boat-house*.

sh may be pronounced as in English.
t and d are soft as in French.

Other consonants appearing in the transliterations may be pronounced as in English.

Diacritical marks have generally not been used in proper names belonging to recent times or in modern and well-known geographical names.

RĀJA-YOGA

Each soul is potentially divine. The goal is to manifest this divinity within by controlling nature: external and internal. Do this either by work, or worship, or psychic control, or philosophy—by one, or more, or all of these—and be free. This is the whole of religion. Doctrines, or dogmas, or rituals, or books, or temples, or forms, are but secondary details.

AUTHOR'S PREFACE

SINCE THE DAWN OF HISTORY various extraordinary phenomena have been recorded as happening amongst human beings. Witnesses are not wanting in modern times to attest such events even in societies living under the full blaze of modern science. The vast mass of such evidence is unreliable, coming as it does from ignorant, superstitious, or fraudulent persons. In many instances the so-called miracles are imitations. But what do they imitate? It is not the sign of a candid and scientific mind to throw overboard anything without proper investigation. Surface scientists, unable to explain the various extraordinary mental phenomena, strive to ignore their very existence. They are therefore more culpable than those who think that their prayers are answered by a being or beings above the clouds, or than those who believe that their petitions will make such beings change the course of the universe. The latter have the excuse of ignorance, or at least of a defective system of education, which has taught them dependence upon such beings, a dependence which has become a part of their degenerate nature. The former have no such excuse.

For thousands of years such phenomena have been studied, investigated, and generalized; the whole ground of the religious faculties of man has been analysed; and the practical result is the science of Rāja-yoga.

Rāja-yoga does not, after the unpardonable manner
of some modern sciences, deny the existence of facts
which are difficult to explain; on the contrary, it
gently, yet in no uncertain terms, tells the superstitious that miracles and answers to prayer and powers
of faith, though true as facts, are not rendered com-
prehensible through superstitious explanations attribut-
ing them to the agency of a being or beings above the
clouds. It declares that each man is only a conduit for
the infinite ocean of knowledge and power that lies
behind mankind. It teaches that desires and wants are
in man, that the power of supply is also in man, and
that wherever and whenever a desire, a want, or a
prayer has been fulfilled, it was out of this infinite
magazine that the fulfilment came, and not from any
supernatural being. The idea of supernatural beings
may rouse to a certain extent the power of action in
man, but it also brings spiritual decay. It brings dependence; it brings fear; it brings superstition. It
degenerates into a horrible belief in the natural weakness of man. There is no supernatural, says the yogi,
but there are in nature gross manifestations and subtle
manifestations. The subtle are the causes, the gross the
effects. The gross can be easily perceived by the senses;
not so the subtle. The practice of rāja-yoga will lead
to the acquisition of the subtle perceptions.

All the orthodox systems of Indian philosophy have
one goal in view: the liberation of the soul through
perfection. The method is yoga. The word *yoga* covers
an immense ground. Both the Sāmkhya and the
Vedānta schools point to yoga in some form or other.

The subject of the present book is that form of yoga

known as Rāja-yoga.[1] The aphorisms of Patanjali are the highest authority on Rāja-yoga and form its textbook. The other philosophers, though occasionally differing from Patanjali in some philosophical points, have, as a rule, accorded to his method of practice a decided consent. The first part of this book comprises several lectures delivered by the present writer to his classes in New York. The second part is a rather free translation of the *Aphorisms (Sutras)* of Patanjali, with a running commentary. An effort has been made to avoid technicalities as far as possible, and to keep to the free and easy style of conversation. In the first part some simple and specific directions are given for students who want to practise; but all such are especially and earnestly warned that, with few exceptions, Rāja-yoga can be safely learnt only by direct contact with a teacher. If these conversations succeed in awakening a desire for further information on the subject, the teacher will not be wanting.

The system of Patanjali is based upon the system of Sāmkhya, the points of difference being very few. The two most important differences are, first, that Patanjali admits the Personal God in the form of the First Teacher, while the only God that Sāmkhya concedes is a nearly perfected being, temporarily in charge

[1] Throughout this volume the editor has followed the policy of spelling *Rāja-yoga* with a capital *r* when the word refers to the well-known system of Yoga philosophy, and with a small *r* when it denotes the spiritual discipline generally known as yoga. But in practice it has not always been possible to maintain this distinction. The word *Yoga*, too, has been spelt with capital *y* and small *y* to denote the Yoga philosophy and the yogic discipline respectively.

of a cycle of creation. Second, a yogi holds the **mind** to be equally all-pervading as the Soul, or Purusha, and Sāmkhya does not.

VIVEKANANDA

INTRODUCTION

ALL OUR KNOWLEDGE is based upon experience. What we call inferential knowledge, in which we go from the particular to the general or from the general to the particular, has experience as its basis. In what are called the exact sciences people easily find the truth, because it appeals to the specific experiences of every human being. The scientist does not ask you to believe in anything blindly; but he has got certain results, which have come from his own experiences, and when, reasoning on them, he wants us to believe in his conclusions, he appeals to some universal experience of humanity. In every exact science there is a basis which is common to all humanity, so that we can at once see the truth or the fallacy of the conclusions drawn therefrom. Now, the question is: Has religion any such basis or not? I shall have to answer the question both in the affirmative and in the negative.

Religion, as it is generally taught all over the world, is found to be based upon faith and belief, and in most cases consists only of different sets of theories; and that is why we find religions quarrelling with one another. These theories, again, are based upon belief. One man says there is a great Being sitting above the clouds and governing the whole universe, and he asks me to believe that solely on the authority of his assertion. In the same way I may have my own ideas, which I am asking others to believe; and if they ask for a reason, I cannot give them any. This is why religion and religious philosophy have a bad name nowadays. Every educated man seems to say: "Oh, these religions are only bundles of theories without any standard to judge them by, each man preaching his own pet ideas." Nevertheless there is a basis of universal belief in religion, governing all the different theories and all the varying ideas of different sects in different countries. Going to this basis, we find that they too are based upon universal experiences.

In the first place, if you analyse the various religions of the world, you will find that they are divided into two classes: those with a book and those without a book. Those with a book are stronger and have a larger number of followers. Those without books have mostly died out, and the few new ones have very small followings. Yet in all of them we find one consensus of opinion: that the truths they teach are the results of the experiences of particular persons. The Christian asks you to believe in his religion, to believe in Christ and to believe in him as the Incarnation of God, to believe in a God, in a soul, and in a better state of that soul. If I ask him for the reason, he says that he believes in them. But if you go to the fountainhead of Christianity, you will find that it is based upon experience. Christ said that he saw God, the disciples said that they felt God, and so forth. Similarly, in Buddhism, it is Buddha's experience. He experienced certain truths, saw them, came in contact with them, and preached them to the world. So with the Hindus:

in their books the writers, who are called rishis, or sages, declare that they have experienced certain truths, and these they preach.

Thus it is clear that all the religions of the world have been built upon that one universal and adamantine foundation of all our knowledge—direct experience. The teachers all saw God; they all saw their own souls, they saw their souls' future and their eternity; and what they saw they preached. Only there is this difference: By most of these religions, especially in modern times, a peculiar claim is made, namely, that these experiences are impossible at the present day; they were possible only to a few men, who were the founders of the religions that subsequently bore their names. At the present time these experiences have become obsolete, and therefore we now have to take these religions on faith.

This I entirely deny. If there has been one experience in this world in any particular branch of knowledge, it absolutely follows that that experience has been possible millions of times before and will be repeated eternally. Uniformity is the rigorous law of nature: what once happened can happen always.

The teachers of the science of Rāja-yoga, therefore, declare not only that religion is based upon the experiences of ancient times, but also that no man can be religious until he has had the same experiences himself. Rāja-yoga is the science which teaches us how to get these experiences. It is not much use to talk about religion until one has felt it. Why is there so much disturbance, so much fighting and quarrelling, in the name of God? There has been more bloodshed in the

name of God than for any other cause, because people
never went to the fountainhead; they were content to
give only a mental assent to the customs of their forefathers, and wanted others to do the same. What right
has a man to say that he has a soul if he does not feel
it, or that there is a God if he does not see Him? If
there is a God we must see Him; if there is a soul we
must perceive it; otherwise it is better not to believe.
It is better to be an outspoken atheist than a hypo-
crite.

The modern idea, on the one hand, with the
"learned" is that religion and metaphysics and all
search after a Supreme Being are futile; on the other
hand, with the semi-educated the idea seems to be
that these things really have no basis, their only value
consisting in the fact that they furnish a strong motive
power for doing good to the world. If men believe in
a God, they may become good and moral, and so make
good citizens. We cannot blame them for holding such
ideas, seeing that all the teaching these men get is
simply to believe in an eternal rigmarole of words,
without any substance behind them. They are asked
to live upon words. Can they do it? If they could, I
should not have the least regard for human nature.
Man wants truth, wants to experience truth for himself. When he has grasped it, realized it, felt it within
his heart of hearts, then alone, declare the Vedas, will
all doubts vanish, all darkness be scattered, and all
crookedness be made straight. "Ye children of immortality, even those who live in the highest sphere,
the way is found. There is a way out of all this dark-

ness, and that is by perceiving Him who is beyond all darkness. There is no other way."

The science of Rāja-yoga proposes to put before humanity a practical and scientifically worked out method of reaching this truth. In the first place, every science must have its own method of investigation. If you want to become an astronomer, and sit down and cry, "Astronomy! astronomy!" you will never become one. It is the same with chemistry. A certain method must be followed. You must go to a laboratory, take different substances, mix them, examine them, experiment with them; and out of that will come a knowledge of chemistry. If you want to be an astronomer you must go to an observatory, take a telescope, and study the stars and planets. And then you will become an astronomer. Each science must have its own methods. I could preach you thousands of sermons, but they would not make you religious until you followed the method. This truth has been preached by sages of all countries, of all ages, by men pure and unselfish who had no motive but to do good to the world. They all declare that they have found certain truths higher than what the senses can bring us, and they invite verification. They ask us to take up the discipline and practise honestly. Then, if we do not find this higher truth, we shall have the right to say that there is no truth in the claim; but before we have done that, we are not rational in denying the truth of their assertions. So we must work faithfully, using the prescribed methods, and light will come.

In acquiring knowledge we make use of generalization, and generalization is based upon observation. We first observe facts, then generalize, and then draw conclusions or formulate principles. The knowledge of the mind, of the internal nature of man, of thought, can never be had until we have first developed the power of observing what is going on within. It is comparatively easy to observe facts in the external world, for many instruments have been invented for the purpose; but in the internal world we have no instrument to help us. Yet we know that we must observe in order to have a real science. Without proper analysis any science will be hopeless, mere theorizing; and that is why the psychologists have been quarrelling among themselves since the beginning of time, except those few who found out the means of observation.

The science of Rāja-yoga proposes, in the first place, to give us such a means of observing the internal states. The instrument is the mind itself. The power of attention, when properly guided and directed towards the internal world, will analyse the mind and illumine facts for us. The powers of the mind are like rays of light dissipated; when they are concentrated they illumine. This is our only means of knowledge. Everyone is using it, both in the external and in the internal world; but, for the psychologist, the same minute observation has to be directed to the internal world which the scientific man directs to the external; and this requires a great deal of practice. From childhood onward we have been taught to pay attention only to things external, but never to things internal; hence most of us have nearly lost the faculty of observing the internal mechanism. To turn the mind, as it were, inside, stop it from going outside, and then to concentrate all its powers and throw them upon the mind itself, in order that it may know its own nature, analyse itself, is very hard work. Yet that is the only way to anything which will be like a scientific approach to the subject.

What is the use of such knowledge? In the first place, knowledge itself is the highest reward of knowledge, and secondly, there is also utility in it. It will take away all our misery. When, by analysing his own mind, a man comes face to face, as it were, with something which is never destroyed, something which is, by its own nature, eternally pure and perfect, he will no more be miserable, no more be unhappy. All misery comes from fear, from unsatisfied desire. When a man finds that he never dies, he will then have no more fear of death. When he knows that he is perfect, he will have no more vain desires. And both these causes being absent, there will be no more misery; there will be perfect bliss, even in this body.

There is only one method by which to attain this knowledge, and that is concentration. The chemist in his laboratory concentrates all the energies of his mind into one focus and throws them upon the materials he is analysing, and thus finds out their secrets. The astronomer concentrates all the energies of his mind and projects them through his telescope upon the skies; and the stars, the sun, and the moon give up their secrets to him. The more I can concentrate my thoughts on the matter on which I am talking to you, the more light I can throw upon it. You are listening to me, and the more you concentrate your thoughts, the more clearly you will grasp what I have to say.

How has all the knowledge in the world been gained but by the concentration of the powers of the mind? The world is ready to give up its secrets if we only know how to knock, how to give it the necessary blow. The strength and force of the blow come through concentration. There is no limit to the power of the human mind. The more concentrated it is, the more power is brought to bear on one point. That is the secret.

It is easy to concentrate the mind on external things; the mind naturally goes outward. But it is not so in religion or psychology or metaphysics, where the subject and the object are one. The object is internal: the mind itself is the object. It is necessary to study the mind itself; the mind studies the mind. We know that there is a power of the mind called reflection. I am talking to you; at the same time I am standing aside, like a second person, and knowing and hearing what I am saying. You work and think at the same time, while a portion of your mind stands by and sees what you are thinking. The powers of the mind should be concentrated and turned back upon it; and as the darkest places reveal their secrets before the penetrating rays of the sun, so will the concentrated mind penetrate into its own innermost secrets. Thus we shall come to the basis of belief, to the real religion. We shall perceive for ourselves whether or not we have souls, whether or not life lasts for five minutes or for eternity, whether or not there is a God. All this will be revealed to us.

This is what Rāja-yoga proposes to teach. The goal

of all its teaching is to show how to concentrate the mind; then how to discover the innermost recesses of our own minds; then how to generalize their contents and form our own conclusions from them. It never asks what our belief is—whether we are deists, or atheists, whether Christians, Jews, or Buddhists. We are human beings, and that is sufficient. Every human being has the right and the power to seek religion; every human being has the right to ask the reason why and to have his question answered by himself—if he only takes the trouble.

So far, then, we see that in the study of Rāja-yoga no faith or belief is necessary. Believe nothing until you find it out for yourself—that is what it teaches us. Truth requires no prop to make it stand. Do you mean to say that the facts of our awakened state require any dreams or imaginings to prove them? Certainly not. The study of Rāja-yoga takes a long time and constant practice. A part of this practice is physical, but in the main it is mental. As we proceed we shall find how intimately the mind is connected with the body. If we believe that the mind is simply a finer part of the body, and that the mind acts upon the body, then it stands to reason that the body must react upon the mind. If the body is sick, the mind becomes sick also. If the body is healthy, the mind remains healthy and strong. When one is angry, the mind becomes disturbed; and when the mind is disturbed, the body also becomes disturbed. With the majority of mankind the mind is greatly under the control of the body, their minds being very little developed. The vast mass of humanity is very little removed from the animals; for in many

instances their power of control is little higher than
that of the animals. We have very little command of
our minds. Therefore to acquire that command, to get
that control over body and mind, we must take certain
physical helps; when the body is sufficiently controlled
we can attempt the manipulation of the mind. By
manipulating the mind, we shall be able to bring it
under our control, make it work as we like, and compel
it to concentrate its powers as we desire.

According to the rāja-yogi, the external world is but
the gross form of the internal, or subtle. The fine is
always the cause, and the gross, the effect. So the
external world is the effect, and the internal, the cause.
Therefore the external forces are simply the grosser
parts of that of which the internal forces are the finer.
The man who has discovered and learnt how to manipulate the internal forces will get the whole of
nature under his control. The yogi proposes to himself
no less a task than to master the whole universe, to
control the whole of nature. He wants to arrive at
the point where what we call nature's laws will have
no influence over him, where he will be able to go
beyond them all. He will be the master of the whole
of nature, internal and external. The progress and
civilization of the human race simply mean controlling
nature.

Different races take to different processes of controlling nature. Just as in the same society some individuals want to control external nature, and others
internal, so, amongst races, some want to control external nature, and others internal. Some say that by
controlling internal nature we control everything;

others, that by controlling external nature we control everything. In the end both are right, because in nature you will not find any such division as internal or external. These are fictitious limitations that never existed. The externalists and the internalists are destined to meet at the same point, when both reach the limits of their knowledge. Just as a physicist, when he pushes his knowledge to its limits, finds that his knowledge melts into metaphysics, so a metaphysician finds that what he calls mind and matter are but apparent distinctions, which will ultimately disappear.

The end and aim of all science is to find the Unity, the One, out of which the manifold is manufactured, the One appearing as many. Rāja-yoga proposes to start from the internal world, study internal nature, and through that, control the whole—both internal and external. It is a very old attempt. India has been its special stronghold, but it has also been attempted by other nations. In Western countries it was regarded as occultism, and people who wanted to practise it were either burnt or killed as witches and sorcerers. In India, for various reasons, it fell into the hands of persons who destroyed ninety per cent of the knowledge and tried to make a great secret of the remainder. In modern times, in the West, one finds many so-called teachers, but these are worse than those of India, because the latter knew something, while these modern exponents know nothing.

Anything that is secret and mysterious in this system of Yoga should be at once rejected. The best guide in life is strength. In religion, as in all other matters, discard everything that weakens you; have nothing to do with it. Mystery-mongering weakens the human brain. It has wellnigh destroyed Yoga, one of the grandest of sciences. From the time it was discovered, more than four thousand years ago, Yoga was perfectly delineated, formulated, and preached in India. It is a striking fact that the more modern the commentator, the greater the mistakes he makes, while the more ancient the writer, the more rational he is. Most of the modern writers talk of all sorts of mysteries. Thus Yoga fell into the hands of a few persons who made it a secret, instead of letting the full blaze of daylight and reason fall upon it. They did so that they might have the powers to themselves.

In the first place there is no mystery in what I shall teach. What little I know I will tell you. So far as I can reason it out I will do so; but as to what I do not know, I will simply tell you what the books say. It is wrong to blindly believe. You must exercise your own reason and judgement; you must learn from experience whether these things happen or not. Just as you would take up any other science, exactly in the same manner you should take up this science for study. There is neither mystery nor danger in it. So far as it is true it ought to be preached in the public streets in broad daylight. Any attempt to mystify these things is productive of great danger.

Before proceeding farther, I will tell you a little of the Sāmkhya philosophy, upon which the whole of Rāja-yoga is based. According to the Sāmkhya philosophy, the genesis of perception is as follows: The impressions of external objects are carried by the outer instruments to their respective brain centres, or organs;

the organs carry the impressions to the mind; the mind, to the determinative faculty; from this the Purusha, the Soul, receives them, when perception results. Next the Purusha gives the order back to the motor centres to do the needful. With the exception of the Purusha, all of these are material; but the mind is much finer matter than the external instruments. That material of which the mind is composed becomes grosser and forms the tanmātras. These become still more gross and form external matter. That is the psychology of Sāmkhya. So between the intellect and the gross matter outside there is only a difference in degree. The Purusha is the only thing which is intelligent. The mind is an instrument, as it were, in the hands of the Soul, through which the Soul perceives external objects.

The mind is constantly changing—running from one object to another. Sometimes it attaches itself to several organs, sometimes to one, and sometimes to none. For instance, if I listen to the clock with great attention, I may not see anything although my eyes are open, showing that the mind was not attached to the organ of vision while it was to the organ of hearing. The mind sometimes attaches itself to all the organs simultaneously. But again, it has the reflexive power of looking back into its own depths. This power the yogi wants to attain; by concentrating the powers of the mind and turning them inward, he seeks to know what is happening inside. There is in this no question of belief; it is the result of the analysis made by certain philosophers. Modern physiologists tell us that the eyes are not the organ of vision, but that the organ is in one of the nerve centres of the brain, and so with all the senses. They also tell us that these centres are formed of the same material as the brain itself. Sāmkhya also tells us the same thing. The former is a statement on the physical side, and the latter on the psychological side; yet both are the same.

Our field of research lies beyond this. The yogi proposes to attain that fine state of perception in which he can perceive all the different mental states. There must be mental perception of all of them. One can perceive how, as soon as an external organ comes in contact with an object, there arises a sensation, how the sensation is carried by a particular nerve to the nerve centre, how the mind receives it, how it is presented to the determinative faculty, and how this last conveys it to the Purusha. All these different steps are to be observed, one by one. As each science requires certain preparations and has its own method, which must be followed before it can be understood, so it is with Rāja-yoga.

Certain regulations as to food are necessary: we must use that food which brings us the purest state of mind. If you go to a menagerie you will find this demonstrated at once. You see the elephants: huge animals, but calm and gentle; and if you go towards the cages of the lions and tigers you find them restless —showing how much difference has been made by food. All the forces that are working in the body have been produced out of food; we see that every day. If you begin to fast, first your body will get weak, the physical forces will suffer. Then, after a few days, the mental forces will suffer also: first memory fails; then comes a point when you are not able to think, much less to pursue any course of reasoning. We have there-fore to take care what sort of food we eat at the begin-ning; and when we have got strength enough, when our practice is well advanced, we need not be so care-ful in this respect. While the plant is growing it must be hedged round, lest it should be injured; but when it becomes a tree the hedges are taken away; it is then strong enough to withstand all assaults.

A yogi must avoid the two extremes of luxury and austerity. He must not fast or torture his flesh. He who does so, says the Gitā, cannot be a yogi; he who fasts, he who keeps awake, he who sleeps much, he who works too much, he who does no work—none of these can be a yogi.

THE FIRST STEPS

Rāja-yoga is divided into eight steps. The first is
yama, which consists of non-killing, truthfulness,
non-stealing, continence, and non-receiving of gifts.
Next is niyama, consisting of cleanliness, contentment,
austerity, study, and self-surrender to God. Then come
āsana, or posture; prānāyāma, or control of the prāna;
pratyāhāra, or restraint of the senses from their objects; dhāranā, or fixing the mind on a spot; dhyāna,
or meditation; and samādhi, or superconscious experience. Yama and niyama are moral training, without
which no practice of yoga will succeed. As the yogi
becomes established in these, he will begin to realize
the fruits of his practice; without them it will never
bear fruit. A yogi must not injure anyone by thought,
word, or deed. Mercy must not be for men alone, but
must go beyond and embrace the whole world.

The next step is āsana, posture. A series of exercises,
physical and mental, is to be gone through every day
until certain higher states are reached. Therefore it is
quite necessary that we should find a posture in which
we can remain for a long time. That posture which is
the easiest should be the one chosen. For thinking, a
certain posture may be very easy for one man, while
for another it may be very difficult. We shall find later
on that during the study of these psychological matters
a good deal of activity goes on in the body. Nerve

currents will have to be displaced and given a new channel. New sorts of vibrations will begin; the whole constitution will be remodelled, as it were. But the main part of the activity will lie along the spinal column; so the one thing necessary for the posture is to hold the spinal column free, sitting erect, holding the three parts—the chest, neck, and head—in a straight line. Let the whole weight of these three be supported by the ribs, and then you will have an easy, natural posture with the spine straight. You will easily see that you cannot think very high thoughts with the chest in.

This portion of yoga is a little similar to hatha-yoga, which deals entirely with the physical body, its aim being to make the physical body very strong. We have nothing to do with it here, because its practices are very difficult and cannot be learnt in a day, and, after all, do not lead to much spiritual growth. Many of these practices—such as placing the body in different postures—you will find in the teachings of Delsarte and others. The object in these is physical, not spiritual. There is not one muscle in the body over which a man cannot establish perfect control: the heart can be made to stop or go on at his bidding, and each part of the organism can be similarly con-trolled.

The result of hatha-yoga is simply to make men live long; health is the chief idea, the one goal of the hatha-yogi. He is determined not to fall sick, and he never does. He lives long. A hundred years is nothing to him; he is quite young and fresh when he is one hundred and fifty, without one hair turned grey. But

that is all. A banyan tree lives sometimes five thousand
years, but it is a banyan tree and nothing more. So
if a man lives long, he is only a healthy animal. But
one or two ordinary lessons of the hatha-yogis are very
useful. For instance, some of you may find it a good
thing for headaches to drink cold water through the
nose as soon as you get up in the morning; the whole
day your brain will feel very cool, and you will never
catch cold. It is very easy to do: put your nose into
the water, draw it up through the nostrils, and make a
pump action in the throat.

After one has learnt to have a firm, erect seat, one
has to perform, according to certain schools, a practice
called the purification of the nerves. This part has
been rejected by some as not belonging to Rāja-yoga;
but since so great an authority as the commentator
Śankarāchārya advises it, I think it fitting that it should
be mentioned, and I will quote his own directions from
his commentary on the *Śvetāśvatara Upanishad:* "The
mind whose dross has been cleared away by prānāyāma
becomes fixed in Brahman; therefore prānāyāma is
taught. First the nerves are to be purified; then comes
the power to practise prānāyāma. Stopping the right
nostril with the thumb, draw in air through the left
nostril according to capacity; then, without any inter-
val, eject the air through the right nostril, closing the
left one. Again inhaling through the right nostril according to capacity, eject through the left. Practising
this three or five times at four periods of the day—
before dawn, during midday, in the evening, and at
midnight—one attains purity of the nerves in fifteen
days or a month. Then begins prānāyāma."

Practice is absolutely necessary. You may sit down and listen to me by the hour every day, but if you do not practise, you will not get one step farther. It all depends on practice. We never understand these things until we experience them. We have to see and feel them for ourselves. Simply listening to explanations and theories will not do.

There are several obstructions to practice. The first obstruction is an unhealthy body; if the body is not fit, the practice will be obstructed. Therefore we have to keep the body in good health; we have to take care about what we eat and drink, and what we do. Always use a mental effort, what is usually called Christian Science, to keep the body strong. That is all; nothing further about the body. We must not forget that health is only a means to an end. If health were the end, then we would be like animals; animals rarely become unhealthy.

The second obstruction is doubt. We always feel doubtful about things we do not see. Man cannot live upon words, however he may try. So doubt comes to us as to whether there is any truth in these things or not; even the best of us will doubt sometimes. With practice, within a few days, a little glimpse will come, enough to give one encouragement and hope. As a certain commentator on Yoga philosophy says: "When one proof is obtained, however little that may be, it will give us faith in the whole teaching of Yoga." For instance, after the first few months of practice you will begin to find you can read another's thoughts; they will come to you in picture form. Perhaps you will hear something happening at a long distance when you concentrate your mind with a wish to hear. These glimpses will come, by little bits at first, but enough to give you faith and strength and hope. For instance, if you concentrate your thoughts on the tip of your nose, in a few days you will begin to smell a most wonderful fragrance, which will be enough to show you that there are certain mental perceptions which one can experience without the contact of physical objects. But we must always remember that these are only the means; the aim, the end, the goal, of all this training is liberation of the soul. Absolute control of nature. and nothing short of it, must be the goal. We must be the masters, and not the slaves, of nature; neither body nor mind must be our master, nor must we forget that the body is ours, and not we the body's.

A god and a demon went to learn about the Self from a great sage. They studied with him for a long time. At last the sage told them, "You yourselves are the Being you are seeking." Both of them thought that their bodies were the Self. The demon went back to his people quite satisfied and said, "I have learnt everything that was to be learnt: eat, drink, and be merry; we are the Self; there is nothing beyond us." The demon was ignorant by nature; so he never inquired any further, but was perfectly contented with the idea that he was God and that by the Self was meant the body.

The god had a purer nature. He at first committed the mistake of thinking, "I, this body, am Brahman; so let me keep it strong and healthy, and well dressed, and give it all sorts of enjoyments." But soon he found out that that could not be the meaning of the sage, their master; there must be something higher. So he came back and said: "Sir, did you teach me that this body was the Self? If so, I see that all bodies die; but the Self should not die." The sage said: "Find it out yourself. Thou art That." Then the god thought that the vital forces which work the body were what he meant by the Self. But after a time he found that if he ate, these vital forces remained strong, but if he starved, they became weak. The god then went back to the sage and said, "Sir, do you mean that the vital forces are the Self?" The sage said: "Find out for yourself. Thou art That." The god returned home once more, thinking that it was the mind, perhaps, that was the Self. But in a short while he saw that his thoughts were extremely various—now good, again bad; the mind was too changeable to be the Self. He went back to the sage and said: "Sir, I do not think that the mind is the Self. Did you mean that?" "No," replied the sage; "thou art That. Find out for yourself." The god went home and at last found the true Self, beyond all thought, one, without birth or death, whom sword cannot pierce or fire burn, whom the air cannot dry or water melt, the beginningless and endless, the immovable, the intangible, the omniscient, the omnipotent Being—neither the body nor the mind, but beyond them both. So he was satisfied; but the poor demon, owing to his fondness for the body, did not get the truth.

This world has a good many of these demoniac natures, but there are some gods too. If one proposes to teach a science to increase the power of sense enjoyment, one finds multitudes ready for it. If one

undertakes to show the supreme goal, one finds few to
listen. Very few have the power to grasp the highest,
fewer still the perseverance to attain to it. But there
are a few who know that even if the body can be
made to live for a thousand years, the result in the
end will be the same. When the forces that hold it
together cease to function, the body must fall. No
man was ever born who could stop his body from
changing. The body is the name of a series of changes.
As in a river the masses of water are changing before
you every moment, and new masses are coming, taking
similar form, so is it with this body. Yet the body
must be kept strong and healthy; it is the best instrument we have.

This human body is the greatest body in the universe, and the human being, the highest being. Man
is higher than all the animals, than all the angels;
none is greater than man. Even the devas, the gods,
will have to come down again and attain to salvation
through a human body. Man alone realizes perfection,
not even the devas. According to the Jews and Mohammedans, God created man after creating the angels
and everything else, and after creating man He asked
the angels to come and salute him, and all did so
except Iblis; so God cursed him and he became Satan.
Behind this allegory is the great truth that this human
birth is the greatest birth we can have. The lower
creation, the animal, is dull and manufactured mostly
out of tamas. Animals cannot have any high thoughts;
nor can the angels or devas attain to direct freedom
without human birth. In human society, in the same
way, too much wealth or too much poverty is a great

impediment to the higher development of the soul. It is from the middle classes that the great ones of the world come. Here the forces are equally adjusted and balanced.

Returning to our subject, we come next to prāṇā-yāma, control of the breathing. What has that to do with concentrating the powers of the mind? The breath is like the fly-wheel of this machine, the body. In a big machine you find the fly-wheel moving first, and that motion is conveyed to finer and finer parts until the most delicate and finest mechanism in the machine is in motion. The breath is that fly-wheel, supplying and regulating the motive power to every-thing in this body.

There was once a minister to a great king. He fell into disgrace. As a punishment, the king ordered him to be shut up in the top of a very high tower. This was done, and the minister was left there to perish. He had a faithful wife, however, who came to the tower at night and called to her husband at the top to know what she could do to help him. He told her to return to the tower the following night and bring with her a long rope, some stout twine, packthread, silk thread, a beetle, and a little honey. Wondering much, the good wife obeyed her husband and brought him the desired articles. The husband directed her to attach the silk thread firmly to the beetle, then to smear its horns with a drop of honey and set it free on the wall of the tower with its head pointing upward. She obeyed all these instructions, and the beetle started on its long journey. Smelling the honey ahead it slowly crept onward, in the hope of reaching the honey, until at last it reached the top of the tower, when the minister grasped the beetle and got possession of the silk thread. He told his wife to tie the other end to the packthread, and after he had drawn up the pack thread, he repeated the process with the stout twine, and lastly with the rope. Then the rest was easy. The minister descended from the tower by means of the rope and made his escape. In this body of ours the motion of the breath is the silk thread; by laying hold of and learning to control it we grasp the packthread of the nerve currents, and from these the stout twine of our thoughts, and lastly the rope of the prāna, controlling which we reach freedom.

We do not know anything about our own bodies. We cannot know. At best we can take a dead body and cut it in pieces; and there are some who can take a live animal and cut it in pieces in order to see what is inside the body. Still that has nothing to do with our own bodies. We know very little about them. Why is that? Because our attention is not discriminating enough to catch the very fine movements that are going on within. We can know of them only when the mind becomes more subtle and enters, as it were, deeper into the body. To get that subtle perception we have to begin with the grosser perceptions. We have to get hold of that which is setting the whole engine in motion; that is the prāna, the most obvious manifestation of which is the breath. Then, along with the breath, we shall slowly enter into the body, and thus be able to find out about the subtle forces, the nerve currents, which are moving all through the body. As soon as we perceive and learn to feel them, we shall begin to get control over them and over the body. The mind is also set in motion by these different nerve currents; so at last we shall reach the state of perfect control over the body and the mind, making both our servants. Knowledge is power. We have to get this power; so we must begin at the beginning, with prāṇāyāma, restraining the prāṇa. This prāṇā-yāma is a long subject, and it will take several lessons to explain it thoroughly. We shall take it up part by part.

We shall gradually see the reasons for each exercise and also what forces in the body are set in motion. All these things will come to us. But it requires constant practice; and the proof will come from practice. No amount of reasoning which I can give you will be proof to you until you have demonstrated it for yourselves. As soon as you begin to feel these currents in motion all over you, doubts will vanish; but it requires hard practice every day. You must practise at least twice every day, and the best times are towards the morning and the evening. When night passes into day, and day into night, a state of relative calmness ensues. The early morning and the early evening are the two periods of calmness. Your body will have a like tendency to become calm at those times. We should take advantage of that natural condition and begin to practise then. Make it a rule not to eat until you have practised; if you do this the sheer force of hunger will break your laziness. In India they teach children never to eat until they have practised or worshipped, and it becomes natural to them after a time; a boy will not feel hungry until he has bathed and practised the disciplines of yoga.

Those of you who can afford it should have a room where you can practise alone. Do not sleep in that room; it must be kept holy. You must not enter the room until you have bathed and are perfectly clean in body and mind. Place flowers in that room always —they are the best surroundings for a yogi—and pictures that are pleasing. Burn incense morning and evening. Have no quarrel or anger or unholy thought in that room. Only allow those persons to enter it who are of the same thought as you. Then gradually there will be an atmosphere of holiness in the room, so that when you are miserable, sorrowful, or doubtful, or when your mind is disturbed, if you then enter the room you will feel inner peace. This was the real idea behind the temple and the church; and in some temples and churches you will find it even now; but in the majority of them this idea has been lost. The fact is that by preserving spiritual vibrations in a place you make it holy. Those who cannot afford to have a room set apart can practise anywhere they like.

Sit in a straight posture. The next thing to do is to send a current of holy thought to all creation. Mentally repeat: "Let all beings be happy; let all beings be peaceful; let all beings be blissful." So do to the east, south, north, and west. The more you practise this, the better you will feel. You will find at last that the easiest way to make ourselves healthy is to see that others are healthy, and the easiest way to make ourselves happy is to see that others are happy. After doing that, those who believe in God should pray—not for money, not for health, nor for heaven. Pray for knowledge and light; every other prayer is selfish. Then the next thing to do is to think that your body is firm, strong, and healthy; for it is the best instrument you have. Think of it as being as strong as adamant, and that with the help of this body you will cross the ocean of life. Freedom is never to be reached by the weak; throw away all weakness. Tell your body that it is strong, tell your mind that it is strong, and have unbounded faith and hope in yourself.

PRĀNA

PRĀNĀYĀMA IS NOT, as many think, concerned solely with the breath; breath indeed has very little to do with it. Breathing is only one of the many exercises through which we get to the real prānāyāma. Prānā-yāma means the control of prāna.

According to the philosophers of India, the universe is composed of two entities, one of which they call ākāśa, and the other, prāna. Ākāśa is the all-penetrating existence. Everything that has form, everything that is the result of combination, is evolved out of ākāśa. It is ākāśa that becomes the air, that becomes the liquids, that becomes the solids; it is ākāśa that becomes the sun, the earth, the moon, the stars, the comets; it is ākāśa that becomes the human body, the animal body, the plants, every form that we see, everything that can be sensed, everything that exists. It cannot be perceived; it is so subtle that it is beyond all ordinary perception; it can only be seen when it has become gross and has taken a form. At the beginning of creation there is only ākāśa; at the end of the cycle the solids, the liquids, and the gases all melt into ākāśa again, and the next creation similarly proceeds out of ākāśa.

By what power is ākāśa manufactured into this universe? By the power of prāna. Just as ākāśa is the infinite, omnipresent material of this universe, so is prāna the infinite, omnipresent manifesting power of this universe. At the beginning and at the end of a cycle all tangible objects resolve back into ākāśa, and all the forces in the universe resolve back into prāna. In the next cycle, out of this prāna is evolved everything that we call energy, everything that we call force. It is prāna that is manifesting as motion; it is prāna that is manifesting as gravitation, as magnetism. It is prāna that is manifesting as the actions of the body, as the nerve currents, as thought-force. From thought down to physical force, everything is but the manifestation of prāna. The sum total of all forces in the universe, mental or physical, when resolved back to their original state, is called prāna. "When there was neither aught nor naught, when darkness covered darkness, what existed then? That ākāśa existed without motion." The physical motion of prāna was stopped, but it existed all the same. At the end of a cycle the energies now displayed in the universe quiet down and become potential. At the beginning of the next cycle they start up, strike upon ākāśa, and thus out of ākāśa evolve these various forms; and as ākāśa changes, prāna changes also into all these manifestations of energy. The knowledge and control of prāna is really what is meant by prānāyāma.

This opens to us the door to almost unlimited power. Suppose, for instance, a man understood prāna perfectly and could control it; what power on earth would not be his? He would be able to move the sun and stars out of their places, to control everything in the universe, from the atoms to the biggest suns. This is the end and aim of prānāyāma. When the yogi be-

comes perfect there will be nothing in nature not
under his control. If he orders the gods or the souls
of the departed to come, they will come at his bidding.
All the forces of nature will obey him as slaves. When
the ignorant see these powers of the yogi they call
them miracles.

One peculiarity of the Hindu mind is that it always
inquires first for the highest possible generalization,
leaving the details to be worked out afterwards. The
question is raised in the Vedas: "What is that, knowing which we shall know everything?" Thus all books
and philosophies have been written for the purpose
of demonstrating that one thing by the knowing of
which everything is known. If a man wants to know
this universe bit by bit he must know every individual
grain of sand, which requires infinite time; he cannot
know all of them. Then how can there be any knowledge? How can a man know all through knowing
particulars? The yogis say that behind this particular
manifestation there is a generalization. Behind all particular ideas stands a generalized, abstract principle.
Grasp it and you have grasped everything. Just as this
whole universe has been generalized, in the Vedas,
into that one Absolute Existence, and he who has
grasped that Existence has grasped the whole universe,
so all forces have been generalized into prāna, and he
who has grasped prāna has grasped all the forces of
the universe, mental and physical. He who has controlled prāna has controlled his own mind and all the
minds that exist. He who has controlled prāna has
controlled his body and all the bodies that exist, because prāna is the source of all energy.

How to control prāna is the sole idea of prānā-yāma. All the trainings and exercises in this regard are for that one end. Each man must begin where he stands, must learn how to control the things that are nearest to him. This body is very near to us, nearer than anything in the external universe; and the mind is nearer than the body. But the prāna which is work-ing this mind and body is the nearest. It is a part of the prāna that moves the universe. In the infinite ocean of prāna, this little wave of prāna which repre-sents our own energies, mental and physical, is the nearest to us. If we can succeed in controlling that little wave, then alone can we hope to control the whole of prāna. The yogi who has done this gains perfection; no longer is he under any power. He becomes almost almighty, almost all-knowing.

We see in every country sects that have attempted the control of prāna. In this country there are mind-healers, faith-healers, spiritualists, Christian Scientists, hypnotists, and so on. If we examine these different sects, we shall find at the back of their methods the control of prāna, whether they know it or not. If you boil all their theories down the residuum will be that. It is one and the same force that they are manipulating, only unknowingly. They have stumbled on the dis-covery of a force and are using it unconsciously with-out knowing its nature; but it is the same as what the yogi uses, and it comes from prāna.

The vital force in every being is prāna. Thought is the finest and highest manifestation of this prāna. Conscious thought, again, as we see it, is not the whole of thought. There is also what we call instinct, or unconscious thought, the lowest plane of thought. If a mosquito bites me, my hand will strike it automatically, instinctively. This is one expression of thought. All reflex actions of the body belong to this plane of thought. There is, again, the other plane of thought, the conscious: I reason, I judge, I think, I see the pros and cons of certain things. Yet that is not all. We know that reason is limited. Reason can go only to a certain length; beyond that it cannot reach. The circle within which it runs is very, very limited indeed. Yet at the same time we find that facts rush into this circle, like comets coming into the earth's orbit. It is plain that they come from outside, although our reason cannot go beyond. The causes of these phenomena which intrude into this small circle are outside it. Yogis say that even this cannot be the limit of knowledge; the mind can function on a still higher plane, the superconscious. When the mind has attained that state, which is called samādhi—perfect concentration—it goes beyond the limits of reason and comes face to face with facts which no instinct or reason can ever know. All manipulations of the subtle forces of the body, different manifestations of prāna, give a push to the mind, help it to go up higher and become superconscious, from where it acts.

In this universe there is one continuous substance on every plane of existence. Physically this universe is one: there is no difference between the sun and you. The scientist will tell you that to say otherwise is without meaning. There is no real difference between this table and me: the table is one point in the mass of matter, and I am another point. Each form represents, as it were, one whirlpool in the infinite ocean of matter. The whirlpools are ever changing. Just as in a rushing stream there may be millions of whirlpools, the water in each of which is different every moment, turning round and round for a few seconds and then passing out, replaced by a fresh quantity, so the whole universe is one constantly changing mass of matter, in which all forms of existence are so many whirlpools. A mass of matter enters into one whirlpool, say a human body, stays there for a period, becomes changed, and goes out into another, say an animal body this time, from which again, after a few years, it enters into another whirlpool, perhaps a lump of mineral. There is constant change. Not one body remains the same. There is no such thing as my body or your body, except in words. Of the one huge mass of matter, one point is called a moon, another a sun, another a man, another the earth, another a plant, another a mineral. Not one is constant, but everything is changing, matter eternally forming and disintegrating.

So it is with the inner world. Matter is represented by the ether;[1] when the action of prāna is most subtle, this ether, in a finer state of vibration, will represent the mind, and there it will be still one unbroken mass. If you can create in yourself that subtle vibration, you will see and feel that the whole universe is composed of subtle vibrations. Sometimes certain drugs have the power to take us to a supersensuous state

[1] During the last part of the nineteenth century the concept of ether was much in vogue among certain scientists.

where we can feel those vibrations. Many of you may remember the celebrated experiment of Sir Humphry Davy, when the laughing-gas overpowered him—how, during the lecture, he remained motionless, stupefied, and how, after that, he said that the whole universe was made up of ideas. For the time being the gross vibrations had ceased and only the subtle vibrations, which he called ideas, were present to him. He could see only the subtle vibrations round him; everything had become thought; the whole universe was an ocean of thought, and he and everyone else had become little thought whirlpools.

Thus even in the universe of thought we find unity; and at last, when we get to the Self, we know that that Self can only be one. Beyond the vibrations of matter in its gross and subtle forms, beyond motion, there is but one. Even in manifested motion there is only unity. These facts can no longer be denied. Modern physics has demonstrated that the sum total of the energies in the universe is the same throughout. It has also been proved that this sum total of energy exists in two forms. It becomes potential, unmanifested, and next it becomes manifested as all these various forces; again it goes back to the quiet state, and again it manifests. Thus it goes on evolving and becoming involved through eternity. The control of this prāna, as before noted, is what is called prānāyāma.

As I have already stated, prānāyāma has very little to do with breathing. But the control of the breath is a means to the real practice of prānāyāma. The most obvious manifestation of prāna in the human body is the motion of the lungs. If that stops, as a rule all other manifestations of force in the body will immediately stop. But there are persons who can train themselves in such a manner that the body will live on, even when this motion has stopped. There are some persons who can bury themselves for days and yet live without breathing. To reach the subtle we must take the help of the gross, and slowly travel towards the most subtle until we gain our objective.

Prānāyāma really means controlling the motion of the lungs, and this motion is associated with the breath. Not that the breath produces it; on the contrary, it produces the breath. This motion draws in the air by pump action. Prāna moves the lungs; the movement of the lungs draws in the air. So prānāyāma is not breathing, but controlling that muscular power which moves the lungs. That muscular power which is transmitted through the nerves to the muscles and from them to the lungs, making them move in a certain manner, is the prāna we have to control through the practice of prānāyāma. When this prāna has become controlled, then we shall immediately find that all the other actions of prāna in the body will slowly come under control. I myself have seen men who have controlled almost every muscle of the body —and why not? If I can control certain muscles, why not every muscle and nerve of the body? What is impossible about that? At present we have lost that control and the motion has become automatic. We cannot move the ears at will, but we know that animals can. We do not have that power because we do not exercise it.

Again, we know that motion which has become

latent can be made manifest. By hard work and practice certain motions of the body which are beyond
our control can be brought under perfect control. Reasoning in this manner, we find that it is not at all impossible, but on the contrary very probable, that each
part of the body can be brought under perfect control.
This the yogi does through prānāyāma.

Perhaps some of you have read that in prānāyāma,
when drawing in the breath, you must fill your whole
body with prāna. In the English translation the word
prāna is given as breath, and you are inclined to ask
how that is to be done. The fault is with the trans-
lator. Every part of the body can be filled with prāna,
the vital force; and when you are able to do that, you
can control the whole body. All the sickness and
misery felt in the body will be perfectly controlled.
Not only so, but you will be able to control another's
body. Everything is infectious in this world—good or
bad. If your body is in a certain state of tension, it
will have a tendency to produce the same tension in
others. If you are strong and healthy, those who live
near you will also have a tendency to become strong
and healthy; but if you are sick and weak, those
around you will have a tendency to become the same.
In the case of one man's trying to heal another, the
first step is simply to transfer his own health to the
other. This is the primitive sort of healing. Consciously or unconsciously, health can be transmitted.
A very strong man, living with a weak man, will
make him feel a little stronger, whether he knows it
or not. When consciously done this action becomes
quicker and better. Next come those cases in which a

person, though he may not be very healthy himself, yet can bring health to another. The first man, in such a case, has a little more control over his prāna, and for the time being can rouse his prāna to a certain state of vibration and transmit it to another person.

There have been cases where this process has been carried on at a distance. But in reality there is no distance which admits of gaps. Where is the distance with such gaps? Is there any gap between you and the sun? There is a continuous mass of matter, the sun being one part, and you another. Is there a gap between one part of a river and another? If not, then why cannot force travel? There is no reason why it cannot. Cases of healing from a distance are perfectly true. Prāna can be transmitted to a very great distance; but for one genuine case there are hundreds of frauds. This process of healing is not so easy as it is thought to be. In the most ordinary cases of such healing you will find that the healers simply take advantage of the naturally healthy state of the human body. An allopath comes and treats cholera patients and gives them his medicines; the homoeopath comes and gives his medicines, and cures perhaps more than the allopath cures, because the homoeopath does not disturb his patients, but allows nature to deal with them. The faith-healer cures still more, because he brings the strength of his mind to bear upon the patient and rouses, through faith, his dormant prāna.

There is a mistake constantly made by faith-healers; they think that faith directly heals a man. But faith alone does not do all the healing. There are diseases where the worst symptom is that the patient never thinks that he has the disease. That tremendous faith of the patient is itself a symptom of the disease and usually indicates that he will die quickly. In such a case the principle that faith cures does not apply. If faith alone cured, these patients also would be cured. It is prāna that really does the curing. The pure-souled man who has controlled his prāna has the power to bring it into a certain state of vibration which can be conveyed to others, arousing in them a similar vibration. You see that in our everyday actions. I am talking to you. What am I trying to do? I am, in reality, bringing my mind to a certain state of vibration, and the more I succeed in bringing it to that state, the more you will be affected by what I say. All of you know that the day I am more enthusiastic, you enjoy the lecture more, and when I am less enthusiastic you feel a lack of interest.

The world-movers, endowed with gigantic will-power, can bring their prāna into a high state of vibration; and it is so great and powerful that it affects others in a moment, and thousands are drawn towards them, and half the world think as they do. The great prophets of the world had the most wonderful control of their prāna, which gave them tremendous will-power; they had brought their prāna to the highest state of vibration, and this is what gave them power to sway the world. All manifestations of power arise from this control. Men may not know the secret, but this is the explanation.

Sometimes in your own body the supply of prāna gravitates more or less to one part; the balance is disturbed, and when the balance of prāna is disturbed, what we call disease is produced. To take away the superfluous prāna, or to supply the prāna that is wanting, will be to cure the disease. To perceive when there is more or less prāna in one part of the body than there should be is also a part of prānāyāma. The perception will be so subtle that the mind will feel that there is less prāna in the toe or the finger than there should be and will possess the power to supply it. These are among the various functions of prānāyāma. They have to be learnt slowly and gradually; and as you see, the whole scope of Rāja-yoga is really to teach the control and direction of prāna in different ways. When a man has concentrated his energies he masters the prāna that is in his body. When a man is meditating he is also controlling his prāna.

In an ocean there are huge waves, like mountains, then smaller waves, and still smaller, down to little bubbles; but back of all these is the infinite ocean. The ocean is connected with the bubble at one end, and with the huge wave at the other end. One man may be a gigantic wave, and another a little bubble, but each is connected with that infinite ocean of energy which is the common birthright of every being that exists. Wherever there is life, the storehouse of infinite energy is behind it. Starting as some fungus, some very minute, microscopic bubble, and all the time drawing from that infinite storehouse of energy, a form changes slowly and steadily, until, in the course of time, it becomes a plant, then an animal, then a man, and ultimately God. This is attained through millions of aeons. But what is time? An increase of speed, an increase of struggle, is able to bridge the gulf of time.

That which naturally takes a long time to accomplish
can be shortened by the intensity of the action, says
the yogi. A man may go on slowly drawing in this
energy from the infinite mass that exists in the
universe, and perhaps he will require a hundred
thousand years to become a deva, and then perhaps
five hundred thousand years to become still higher,
and perhaps five million years to become perfect.
Given rapid growth, the time will be lessened. Why
is it not possible, with sufficient effort, to reach this
very perfection in six years or six months? There is
no limit. Reason shows that. If an engine, with a
certain amount of coal, runs two miles an hour, it will
run the distance in less time with a greater supply of
coal. Similarly, why should not the soul, by intensifying its action, attain perfection in this very life?
All beings will at last attain to that goal, we know.
But who cares to wait all these millions of aeons? Why
not reach it immediately, even in this body, in this
human form? Why should I not get that infinite
knowledge, infinite power, now?

The ideal of the yogi, the whole science of Yoga, is
directed to the end of teaching men how, by intensifying the power of assimilation, to shorten the
time for reaching perfection instead of slowly ad-
vancing from point to point and waiting until the
whole human race has become perfect. All the great
prophets, saints, and seers of the world—what did
they do? In one span of life they lived the whole life
of humanity, traversed the whole length of time that
it takes an ordinary man to come to perfection. In one

life they perfected themselves; they had no thought for anything else, never lived a moment for any other idea, and thus the way was shortened for them. This is what is meant by concentration: intensifying the power of assimilation, thus shortening the time. Rāja-yoga is the science which teaches us how to gain the power of concentration.

What has prānāyāma to do with spiritualism? Spiritualism is also a manifestation of prānāyāma. If it be true that the departed spirits exist, only we cannot see them, it is quite probable that there are hundreds and millions of them about us that we can neither see, feel, nor touch. We may be continually passing and repassing through their bodies, and they do not see or feel us. It is plane within plane, universe within universe. We have five senses, and we represent prāna in a certain state of vibration. All beings in the same state of vibration will see one another; but if there are beings who represent prāna in a higher state of vibration, they will not be seen. We may increase the intensity of a light until we cannot see it at all, but there may be beings with eyes so powerful that they can see such a light. Again, if its vibrations are very low we do not see a light, but there are animals that can see it, such as cats and owls. Our range of vision is only one plane of the vibrations of prāna. Take the atmosphere, for instance: it is piled up layer on layer, but the layers nearer the earth are denser than those above, and as you go higher the atmosphere becomes finer and finer. Or take the ocean: as you go deeper and deeper the pressure of the water increases, and the animals which live at the bottom of the sea can never come up, or they will be broken into pieces.

Think of the whole universe as an ocean of ether, vibrating under the action of prāna and consisting of plane after plane of varying degrees of vibration. In the more external the vibrations are slower, and nearer the centre they are quicker. Think of the whole thing as a circle, the centre of which is perfection. The farther you move from the centre, the slower are the vibrations. Matter is the outermost plane; next comes mind; and Spirit is the centre. Now, it is clear that those who live on a certain plane of vibration will have the power to recognize each other but will not recognize those above or below them. Yet, just as by the telescope and the microscope we can increase the scope of our vision, similarly by yoga we can bring ourselves to the state of vibration of another plane and thus enable ourselves to see what is going on there.

Suppose this room is full of beings whom we do not see. They represent prāna in a certain state of vibration, while we represent another. Suppose they represent a quick one, and we the opposite. Prāna is the material of which they are composed, as well as we. We are all parts of the same ocean of prāna and we differ only in the rate of vibration. If I can bring myself to the quick vibration, this plane will immediately change for me; I shall not see you any more; they will appear. Some of you, perhaps, know this to be true. All this bringing of the mind into a higher state of vibration is included in one word in Yoga: samādhi. All these states of higher vibration, superconscious vibration of the mind, are indicated by that one word *samādhi;* and the lower states of samādhi give us visions of these supernatural beings. In the highest kind of samādhi we see the real thing, we see the material out of which all these classes of beings are composed. One lump of clay being known, we know all the objects made of clay in the universe.

Thus we see that prānāyāma includes all that is true even of spiritualism. Similarly, you will find that wherever any sect or body of people is trying to discover anything occult, mysterious, or hidden, they are really practising some sort of yoga, attempting to control their prāna. You will find that wherever there is any extraordinary display of power, it is the manifestation of prāna. Even the physical sciences can be included in prānāyāma. What moves the steam-engine? Prāna acting through the steam. What are all these phenomena of electricity and so forth but prāna? What is physical science? The science of prānāyāma by external means. Prāna, manifesting itself as mental power, can only be controlled by mental means. That part of prānāyāma which attempts to control the physical manifestations of prāna by physical means is called physical science, and that part which tries to control the manifestations of prāna as mental force, by mental means, is called Rāja-yoga.

THE PSYCHIC PRĀNA

ACCORDING TO THE YOGIS there are two nerve currents in the spinal column called the Pingalā
and the Idā, and a hollow canal called the Sushumnā
running through the spinal cord. At the lower end of
the canal is what the yogis called the "lotus of the
Kundalini." They describe it as triangular in form. In
it, in the symbolical language of the yogis, there is
coiled up a power called the Kundalini. When the
Kundalini awakes, it tries to force a passage through
this hollow canal; and as it rises step by step, as it
were, layer after layer of the mind opens up and
many different visions and wonderful powers come to
the yogi. When it reaches the brain, the yogi becomes
perfectly detached from the body and mind; the soul
realizes its freedom.

We know that the spinal cord is shaped in a peculiar
manner. If we take the figure eight horizontally (∞),
we see two parts, which are connected in the middle.
Now if you pile up a number of eights, one on top
of another, that will represent the spinal cord. The
left side is the Idā, the right is the Pingalā, and that
hollow canal which runs through the centre of the
spinal cord is the Sushumnā. Where the spinal cord
ends in some of the lumbar vertebrae, a fine fibre
issues downwards, and the canal runs even through
that fibre, only much finer. The canal is closed at

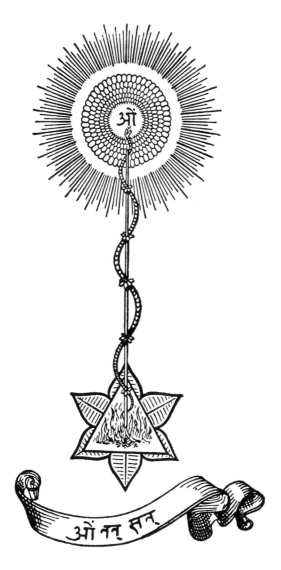

A Symbolic Representation of the Kundalini Rising
through the Different Centres in the Sushumnā
to the Thousand-petalled Lotus in the Brain

the lower end, situated near what is called the sacral plexus, which, according to modern physiology, is triangular in form. The different plexuses that have their centres in the spinal canal can very well stand for the different "lotuses" of the yogi.

The yogi describes several centres, beginning with the Mulādhāra, the basic, and ending with the Sahas- rāra, the thousand-petalled lotus in the brain. So if we take the different plexuses as representing these lotuses, the idea of the yogi can be understood very easily in the language of modern physiology. We know that there are two sorts of actions in the nerve cur- rents: one afferent, and the other efferent; one sen- sory, and the other motor; one centripetal, and the other centrifugal. One carries the sensations to the brain, and the other, from the brain to the outer parts of the body. In the long run these vibrations are all connected with the brain.

There are several other facts which we have to remember in order to clear the way for the explanation which is to come. The spinal cord, at the brain, ends in a sort of bulb in the *medulla,* which is not attached to the brain but floats in a fluid in the brain, so that if there is a blow on the head the force of that blow will be dissipated in the fluid and will not hurt the bulb. This is an important fact to remember. Secondly, we have also to remember that, of all the centres, three are particularly important: the Mulādhāra (the basic), the Sahasrāra (the thousand-petalled lotus in the brain), and the Manipura (the lotus at the navel).

Next we shall take one fact from physics. We all hear of electricity and various other forces connected

with it. What electricity is no one knows, but so far
as it is known, it is a sort of motion. There are various
other motions in the universe. What is the difference
between them and electricity? Suppose that this table
moves and that the molecules which compose this
table are moving in different directions; but if they
are all made to move in the same direction, then this
motion will be electricity. Electricity becomes manifest
when the molecules of a body move in the same direction. If all the air molecules in a room are made to
move in the same direction, that will make a gigantic
battery of electricity of the room.

Another point we must remember—from physiology
—is that the nerve centre which regulates the respiratory system, the breathing system, has a controlling
action over the whole system of nerve currents. Now
we can see why rhythmical breathing is practised. In
the first place, from it comes a tendency of all the
molecules in the body to move in the same direction.
When the mind, by nature distracted, becomes one-
pointed and thus is changed into a strong will, the
nerve currents, too, change into a motion similar to
electricity; for the nerves have been proved to show
polarity under the action of electric currents. This
shows that when the will is transformed into the nerve
currents it changes into something like electricity.
Therefore when all the motions of the body have become perfectly rhythmical, the body becomes a gigantic
battery of will. This tremendous will is exactly what
the yogi wants to acquire. This is, therefore, the
physiological explanation of prāṇāyāma; it tends to
bring a rhythmic action in the body, and helps us,

through the respiratory centre, to control the other centres. The aim of prānāyāma is to rouse the coiled-up power in the Mulādhāra, called the Kundalini.

Everything that we see or imagine or dream, we have to perceive in space. This is the ordinary space, called the mahākāśa, or physical space. When a yogi reads the thoughts of other men or perceives super-sensuous objects, he sees them in another sort of space, called the chittākāśa, the mental space. When perception has become objectless and the Soul shines in Its own nature, it is called the Chidākāśa, or Knowledge space. When the Kundalini is aroused and enters the canal of the Sushumnā, all the perceptions are in the mental space. When it has reached that end of the canal which opens out into the brain, the objectless perception is in the Knowledge space.

Taking the analogy of electricity, we find that man can send a current only along a wire,[1] but nature requires no wires to send her tremendous currents. This proves that the wire is not really necessary; only our inability to dispense with it compels us to use it. Similarly, all the sensations and motions of the body are being sent into the brain, and sent out of it, through these wires of the nerve fibres. The columns of the sensory and motor fibres in the spinal cord are the Idā and Pingalā of the yogis. They are the main channels through which the afferent and efferent currents travel. But why should not the mind send news without any wire or react without any wire? We see this done in nature. The yogi says that if you can do

[1] The reader should remember that this was said before the discovery of wireless telegraphy.

that you have got rid of the bondage of matter. How
can you do it? If you can make the current pass through
the Sushumnā, the canal in the middle of the spinal
column, you have solved the problem. The mind has
made this network of the nervous system, and it has to
break it so that no wires will be required to work
through. Then alone will all knowledge come to us—
no more bondage of the body. That is why it is so important that we should get control of the Sushumnā. If
we can send the mental current through that hollow
canal without any nerve fibres to act as wires, the yogi
says, the problem is solved. And he also says it can be
done. This Sushumnā is in ordinary persons closed
up at the lower extremity; no current comes through
it. The yogi proposes a practice by which it can be
opened and the nerve currents made to travel through
it.

When a sensation is carried to a centre, the centre
reacts. This reaction, in the automatic centres, is followed by motion; in the conscious centres it is followed
first by perception and secondly by motion. All perception is the reaction to action from outside. How,
then, do perceptions in dreams arise? There is then
no action from outside. The sensations must therefore
have been coiled up somewhere. For instance, I see
a city. The perception of that city is from my reaction
to the sensations brought from outside objects comprising that city. That is to say, a certain motion in
the brain molecules has been set up by the motion
in the in-carrying nerves, which, again, are set in
motion by external objects in the city. Now, even
after a long time I can remember the city. Dreams

are exactly the same phenomena, only in a milder form. But whence is the action that set up even the milder form of similar vibrations in the brain? Certainly not from the primary sensations. Therefore it must be that the sensations are coiled up somewhere, and by their action bring out the mild reaction which we call dream perception.

Now, the centre where all these residual sensations are, as it were, stored up, is called the Mulādhāra, the root receptacle, and the coiled-up energy of action is the Kundalini, the "coiled up." It is very probable that the residual motor energy is also stored up in the same centre, since, after deep study or meditation on external objects, the part of the body where the Mulādhāra centre is situated—probably the sacral plexus—gets heated. Now, if this coiled-up energy is roused and made active and then consciously made to travel up the Sushumnā canal, as it acts upon centre after centre, a tremendous reaction will set in. When a minute portion of energy travels along a nerve fibre and causes a reaction from the centres, the perception is either dream or imagination. But when by the power of long internal meditation the vast mass of energy stored up travels along the Sushumnā and strikes the centres, the reaction is tremendous, immensely superior to the reaction of dream or imagination, immensely more intense than the reaction of sense perception. It is supersensuous perception. And when it reaches the metropolis of all sensations, the brain, the whole brain, as it were, reacts, and the result is the full blaze of illumination, the perception of the Self. As this Kundalini force travels from centre to centre, layer after

layer of the mind, as it were, opens up, and the
universe is perceived by the yogi in its fine, or causal,
form. Then alone are the causes of the universe, both
as sensation and as reaction, known as they are; and
hence comes all knowledge. The cause being known,
the knowledge of the effects is sure to follow.

Thus the rousing of the Kundalini is the one and
only way to the attaining of divine wisdom, superconscious perception, realization of the Spirit. The
rousing may come in various ways: through love for
God, through the mercy of perfected sages, or through
the power of the analytic will of the philosopher.
Wherever there has been any manifestation of what is
ordinarily called supernatural power or wisdom, there
a little current of the Kundalini must have found its
way into the Sushumnā. Only, in the vast majority
of such cases, the people had ignorantly stumbled
on some practice which set free a minute portion of
the coiled-up Kundalini. All worship, consciously or
unconsciously, leads to this end. The man who thinks
that he is receiving a response to his prayers does
not know that the fulfilment comes from his own
nature, that he has succeeded, by the mental attitude
of prayer, in waking up a bit of this infinite power
which is coiled up within himself. Thus what men
ignorantly worship under various names, through fear
and tribulation, the yogi declares to the world to be
the real power coiled up in every being, the Mother
of eternal happiness. And Rāja-yoga is the science of
religion, the rationale of all worship, all prayers, forms,
ceremonies, and miracles.

THE CONTROL OF THE PSYCHIC PRĀNA

WE HAVE NOW to deal with the exercises in prāna-yāma. We have seen that the first step, according to the yogis, is to control the motion of the lungs. What we want to do is to feel the finer motions that are going on in the body. Our minds have become externalized and have lost sight of the fine motions inside. If we can begin to feel them, we can also begin to control them. These nerve currents flow all through the body, bringing life and vitality to every muscle; but we do not feel them. The yogi says that we can learn to do so. How? It is by controlling the motion of the lungs. When we have done that for a sufficient length of time we shall be able to control the finer motions in the body.

We now come to the exercises in prānāyāma. Sit upright; the body must be kept straight. The spinal cord, although not attached to the vertebral column, is yet inside it. If you sit crookedly you disturb the spinal cord; so let it be free. Any time that you sit crookedly and try to meditate you do yourself an injury. The three parts of the body—the chest, the neck, and the head—must always be held straight, in one line. You will find that by a little practice this will come to you as easily as breathing. The second thing is to get control of the nerves. We have said that the nerve centre that controls the respiratory

organs has a sort of controlling effect on the other
nerves, and rhythmical breathing is therefore necessary. The way we generally breathe should not be
called breathing at all; it is very irregular. Then there
are some natural differences of breathing between men
and women.

The first lesson is to breathe, in a measured way,
in and out. That will harmonize the system. When
you have practised this for some time, you may repeat
along with your breathing the word *Om,* or any other
sacred word. In India we use certain symbolical words
to measure the periods of inhalation and exhalation,
instead of counting one, two, etc. That is why I advise
you to mentally repeat a sacred word while you practise. Let the word flow in and out with the breath,
rhythmically, and you will find that the whole body
is becoming rhythmical. Then you will enjoy real rest.
Compared with it, sleep is no rest. Once this rest
comes, the most tired nerves will be calmed down
and you will find that you have never before really
rested.

The first effect of this practice is perceived in a
change of expression in one's face. Harsh lines disappear; with calm thought, calmness comes over the face.
Next comes a beautiful voice. I never saw a yogi with
a croaking voice. These signs come after a few months'
practice.

After practising the above-mentioned breathing for a
few days, you should take up a higher one. Slowly fill
the lungs with breath through the left nostril, and at
the same time concentrate the mind on the Idā, the
left nerve current. You are, as it were, sending the

nerve current down the spinal column and striking violently the last plexus, the basic lotus, which is triangular in form, the seat of the Kundalini. Then hold the current there for some time. Next imagine that you are slowly drawing that nerve current, with the breath, through the other side, the Pingalā; then slowly exhale it through the right nostril. This you will find a little difficult. The easiest way is to stop the right nostril with the thumb and then slowly draw in the breath through the left; then close both nostrils with thumb and forefinger, and imagine that you are sending that current down and striking the base of the Sushumnā; then take the thumb off and let the breath out through the right nostril. Next inhale slowly through that nostril, keeping the other closed with the forefinger; then close both, as before.

The way the Hindus practise this would be very difficult for the people of this country, because they do it from their childhood and their lungs are prepared for it. Here it is well to begin with four seconds and slowly increase. Draw in for four seconds, hold in for sixteen seconds, then exhale in eight seconds. This makes one prānāyāma. At the same time think of the basic lotus, triangular in form; concentrate the mind on that centre. The imagination can help you a great deal.

The next exercise is to slowly draw the breath in and then immediately exhale it slowly, and then stop the breath altogether, using the same numbers. The only difference is that in the first case the breath is held in, and in the second, held out. This last is the easier one. The exercise in which you hold the breath

in the lungs must not be practised too much. Do it
only four times in the morning and four times in the
evening. Then you can slowly increase the time and
number. You will find that you have the power to
do so and that you take pleasure in it. So, very carefully and cautiously increase the number, as you feel
that you have the power, to six instead of four. It
may injure you if you practise it irregularly.

Of the three processes for the control of prāna, described above, the first and the last are neither difficult
nor dangerous. The more you practise the first one,
the calmer you will be. Repeat Om as you breathe;
you can practise even while you are sitting at your
work. You will be all the better for it. Some day,
if you practise hard, the Kundalini will be aroused.
For those who practise once or twice a day, just a
little calmness of body and mind will ensue, and a
beautiful voice. Only for those who can go on farther
with it will the Kundalini be aroused. Then the whole
of nature will begin to change and the door of knowledge will open. No more will you need to go to
books for knowledge; your own mind will become your
book, containing infinite knowledge.

I have already spoken of the Idā and Pingalā currents, flowing through either side of the spinal column,
and also of the Sushumnā, the passage through the
centre of the spinal cord. These three are present in
every animal—whatever creature has a spinal column.
But the yogis claim that in ordinary beings the Sushumnā is closed, its action is not evident, while that
of the other two carries power to different parts of the
body.

For the yogi alone the Sushumnā opens. When the current begins to rise through the Sushumnā, we go beyond the senses, and our minds become supersensuous, superconscious; we go beyond even the intellect, where reasoning cannot reach. To open the Sushumnā is the prime object of the yogi. According to him, along the Sushumnā are ranged the centres, or, in the figurative language of Yoga, lotuses. The lowest one is at the bottom of the spinal cord and is called the Mulādhāra, the next higher is called the Svādhisthāna, the third the Manipura, the fourth the Anāhata, the fifth the Viśuddha, the sixth the Ājnā, and the last, which is in the brain, is called the Sahasrāra, or "thousand-petalled." Of these we have to take cognizance just now of two centres only: the lowest, the Mulādhāra, and the highest, the Sahasrāra. All the energy has to be taken up from its seat in the Mulādhāra and brought to the Sahasrāra.

The yogis claim that, of all the energies that are in the human body, the highest is what they call ojas. Now, this ojas is stored up in the brain, and the more ojas a man has, the more powerful he is, the more intellectual, the more spiritually strong. One man may express beautiful thoughts in beautiful language, but cannot impress people. Another man may not be able to give beautiful expression to his thoughts, yet his words charm; every movement of his is powerful. That is the power of ojas.

Now, in every man there is stored up more or less of this ojas. The highest form of all the forces that are working in the body is ojas. You must remember that it is only a question of transformation of one force into another. The same force which is working outside as electricity or magnetism will be changed into inner force; the same force that is working as muscular energy will be changed into ojas. The yogis say that that part of the human energy which is expressed through sexual action and sexual thought, when checked and controlled, easily becomes changed into ojas; and since the Mulādhāra guides these, the yogi pays particular attention to that centre. He tries to convert all his sexual energy into ojas. It is only the chaste man or woman who can create ojas and store it in the brain; that is why chastity has always been considered the highest virtue. A man feels that if he is unchaste, his spirituality goes away; he loses mental vigour and moral stamina. That is why, in all the religious orders in the world which have produced spiritual giants, you will always find absolute chastity insisted upon. That is why there came into existence monks, who gave up marriage. There must be perfect chastity in thought, word, and deed. Without it the practice of rāja-yoga is dangerous and may lead to insanity. If people practise rāja-yoga and at the same time lead an impure life, how can they expect to become yogis?

PRATYĀHĀRA AND DHĀRANĀ

THE NEXT STEP is called pratyāhāra. What is this? You know how perceptions arise. First of all there are the external instruments, then the internal organs, functioning in the body though the brain centres, and last there is the mind. When these join together and attach themselves to some external object, then we perceive it. At the same time it is very difficult to concentrate the mind and attach it to one organ only; the mind is a slave of physical objects.

We hear "Be good," "Be good," "Be good," taught all over the world. There is hardly a child born in any country in the world who has not been told, "Do not steal," "Do not tell a lie"; but nobody tells the child how he can avoid stealing or lying. Talking will not help him. Why should he not become a thief? We do not teach him how not to steal; we simply tell him, "Do not steal." Only when we teach him how to control his mind do we really help him.

All actions, internal and external, occur when the mind joins itself to certain centres, called organs. Willingly or unwillingly people join their minds to the centres, and that is why they do foolish deeds and feel miserable. But if the mind were under control they would not do so. What would be the result of controlling the mind? It then would not join itself to the centres of perception, and naturally feeling and

willing would be under control. It is clear so far. But
is this possible? Certainly it is; you see it practised
in modern times. The faith-healers teach people to
deny misery and pain and evil. Their philosophy is
rather roundabout, but it is a part of yoga upon which
they have somehow stumbled. Where they succeed in
making a person throw off suffering by denying it,
they really use a part of pratyāhāra, for they make
the mind of the person strong enough to ignore the
senses. The hypnotists, in a similar manner, by their
suggestion excite in the patient a sort of morbid pratyāhāra for the time being. So-called hypnotic suggestion
can act only upon a weak mind; and until the opera-
tor, by means of fixed gaze or something else, has
succeeded in putting the mind of the subject in a
sort of passive, morbid condition, his suggestions never
work.

Now, the control of the centres which for a time
is established in a patient, whether by a hypnotist or
by a faith-healer, is reprehensible, because it leads to
ultimate ruin. It is not really controlling the brain
centres by the power of the patient's own will, but it
is, as it were, stunning his mind for a time by sudden
blows which another's will delivers to it. It is not
checking the mad career of a fiery team by means of
reins and muscular strength, but rather by asking
another to deliver heavy blows on the heads of the
horses in order to stun them for a time into gentle-
ness. By each one of these processes the man operated
upon loses a part of his mental energies, till at last
his mind, instead of gaining the power of perfect
control, becomes a shapeless, powerless mass and the

only destination of the patient is the lunatic asylum.

Every attempt at control which is not voluntary, not made with the individual's own will, not only is disastrous but defeats its own end. The goal of each soul is freedom, mastery—freedom from the slavery of matter and thought, mastery of external and internal nature. Instead of leading towards that, every will-current from another, in whatever form it comes, either directly controlling the organs or forcing one to control them while under a morbid condition, only rivets one more link to the already existing heavy chain of the bondage of past thoughts, past superstitions. Therefore beware how you allow yourselves to be acted upon by others. Beware how you unknowingly bring another to ruin. True, some succeed in doing good to many, for a time, by giving a new trend to their propensities; but at the same time they bring ruin to millions by the unconscious suggestions they throw around, rousing in men and women that morbid, passive, hypnotic condition which makes them at last almost soulless.

Whosoever asks anyone to believe blindly, or drags people behind him by the controlling power of his superior will, does an injury to humanity, though he may not intend it. Therefore use your own minds, control body and mind yourselves, and remember that unless you are a diseased person no extraneous will can work upon you. Avoid everyone, however great and good he may be, who asks you to believe blindly.

All over the world there have been dancing and jumping and howling sects, whose influence spreads like infection as they sing and dance and preach;

they too are a sort of hypnotists. They exercise a singular control for the time being over sensitive persons—alas! often, in the long run, to degenerate whole races. Ay, it is healthier for the individual or the race to remain wicked than to be made apparently good by such morbid, extraneous control. One's heart sinks to think of the amount of injury done to humanity by such irresponsible yet well-meaning religious fanatics. They little know that the minds which attain to sudden spiritual upheaval under their suggestions, with music and prayers, are simply making themselves passive, morbid, and powerless and opening themselves to any other suggestion, be it ever so evil. Little do these ignorant, deluded persons dream that, while they are congratulating themselves upon their miraculous power to transform human hearts, which power they think was poured upon them by some Being above the clouds, they are sowing the seeds of future decay, of crime, of lunacy, and of death. Therefore beware of everything that takes away your freedom. Know that it is dangerous and avoid it by all the means in your power.

He who has succeeded in attaching or detaching his mind to or from the centres at will has succeeded in pratyāhāra, which means "gathering towards," checking the outgoing powers of the mind, freeing it from the thraldom of the senses. When we can do this we shall really possess character. Then we shall have taken a long step towards freedom; before that we are mere machines.

How hard it is to control the mind! Well has it been compared to the maddened monkey in the story. There was a monkey, restless by his own nature, as all monkeys are. As if that were not enough, some-one made him drink freely of wine, so that he became still more restless. Then a scorpion stung him. When a man is stung by a scorpion he jumps about for a whole day; so the poor monkey found his condition worse than ever. To complete his misery a demon entered into him. What language can describe the uncontrollable restlessness of the monkey? The human mind is like that monkey. Incessantly active by its own nature, it then becomes drunk with the wine of desire, thus increasing its turbulence. After desire has taken possession, comes the sting of the scorpion of jealousy at the success of others; and last of all the demon of pride enters the mind, making it think itself all-important. How hard to control such a mind!

The first lesson, then, is to sit for some time and let the mind run on. The mind is bubbling up all the time. It is like that monkey jumping about. Let the monkey jump as much as he can; you simply wait and watch. Knowledge is power, says the proverb, and that is true. Until you know what the mind is doing you cannot control it. Give it the rein. Many hideous thoughts may come into it; you will be astonished that it was possible for you to harbour such thoughts; but you will find that each day the mind's vagaries are becoming less and less violent, that each day it is becoming calmer. In the first few months you will find that the mind has a great many thoughts; later you will find that they have somewhat decreased, and in a few more months they will be fewer and fewer, until at last the mind is under perfect control.

But you must patiently practise every day. As long as the steam is there, the engine must run; as long as things are before us, we must perceive them. So a man, to prove that he is not a machine, must demonstrate that he is under the control of nothing. This controlling of the mind and not allowing it to join itself to the centres is pratyāhāra. How is this practised? It is a tremendous work; it cannot be done in a day. Only after a patient, continuous struggle for years can we succeed.

After you have practised pratyāhāra for a time, take the next step, dhāranā, holding the mind to certain points. What is meant by holding the mind to certain points? Forcing the mind to feel certain parts of the body to the exclusion of others. For instance, try to feel only the hand, to the exclusion of other parts of the body. When the chitta, or mind-stuff, is confined and limited to a certain place, it is dhāranā. This dhāranā is of various sorts, and along with it, it is better to have a little play of the imagination. For instance, the mind should be made to think of one point in the heart. That is very difficult; an easier way is to imagine a lotus there. That lotus is full of light—effulgent light. Put the mind there. Or think of the lotus in the brain as full of light, or of the different centres in the Sushumnā mentioned before.

The yogi must always practise. He should try to live alone; the companionship of different sorts of people distracts the mind. He should not speak much, because to speak distracts the mind; not work much, because too much work distracts the mind; the mind cannot be controlled after a whole day's hard work. One observing the above rules becomes a yogi.

Such is the power of yoga that even the least of it will bring a great amount of benefit. It will not hurt anyone but will benefit everyone. First of all, it will calm down nervous excitement, bring peace, enable us to see things more clearly. The temperament will be better and the health will be better. Sound health will be one of the first signs, and a beautiful voice. Defects in the voice will be changed. This will be among the first of the many effects that will come. Those who practise hard will get many other signs. Sometimes there will be sounds, as of a peal of bells heard at a distance, commingling and falling on the ear as one continuous sound. Sometimes things will be seen—little specks of light floating and becoming bigger and bigger; and when these things appear, know that you are progressing fast. Those who want to be yogis and to practise hard must be careful about their diet at first. But those who want only a little practice for an everyday, business sort of life—let them not eat too much; otherwise they may eat whatever they please.

For those who want to make rapid progress and to practise hard a strict diet is absolutely necessary. They will find it advantageous to live only on milk and cereals for some months. As the bodily organization becomes finer and finer, it will be found in the beginning that the least irregularity throws one out of balance. One bit of food more or less will disturb the whole system, until one gets perfect control, and then one will be able to eat whatever one likes. When one begins to concentrate, the dropping of a pin will seem like a thunderbolt going through the brain. As the organs get finer, the perceptions get finer. These are stages through which we have to pass, and all those who persevere will succeed. Give up all argumentation and other distractions. Is there anything in dry, intellectual jargon? It only throws the mind off its balance and disturbs it. The things of the subtler planes have to be realized. Will talking do that? So give up all vain talk. Read only those books which have been written by persons who have had spiritual experiences.

Be like the pearl-oyster. There is a pretty Indian fable to the effect that if it rains when the star Svāti is in the ascendant, and a drop of rain falls into an oyster, that drop becomes a pearl. The oysters know this; so they come to the surface when that star appears, and wait to catch the precious raindrops. When the drops fall into them, quickly the oysters close their shells and dive down to the bottom of the sea, there patiently to develop the raindrops into pearls. You should be like that. First hear, then understand, and then, leaving all distractions, shut your minds to outside influences and devote yourselves to developing the truth within you. There is a danger of frittering away your energies by taking up an idea only for its novelty and then giving it up for another that is newer. Take one thing up and follow it, and see the end of it, and before you have seen the end, do not give it up. He who can become mad with an idea, he alone sees the light. Those who only take a nibble here and a nibble there will never attain any-thing. They may titillate their nerves for a moment, but there it will end. They will be slaves in the hands of nature and will never go beyond the senses.

Those who really want to be yogis must give up, once for all, this nibbling at things. Take up one idea; make that one idea your life. Think of it, dream of it, live on that idea. Let the brain, muscles, nerves, every part of your body, be full of that idea, and just leave all other ideas alone. This is the way to success and this is the way great spiritual giants are produced. Others are mere talking-machines. If we really want to be blessed and make others blessed, we must go deeper.

The first step is not to disturb the mind, not to associate with persons whose ideas are disturbing. All of you know that certain persons, certain places, cer-tain foods, repel you. Avoid them; and those who want to realize the highest must avoid all company, good or bad. Practise hard; whether you live or die does not matter. You have to plunge in and work without thinking of the result. If you are brave enough, in six months you will be a perfect yogi. But those who take up just a bit of it and a little of everything else make no progress. It is of no use simply to take a course of lessons. To those who are full of tamas, ignorant and dull—those whose minds never get fixed on any idea, who only crave for some-thing to amuse them—religion and philosophy are simply objects of entertainment. These are the un-persevering. They hear a talk, think it very nice, and then go home and forget all about it. To succeed you must have tremendous perseverance, tremendous will. "I will drink the ocean," says the persevering soul, "and at my will mountains will crumble." Have that sort of energy, that sort of will, work hard, and you will reach the goal.

DHYĀNA AND SAMĀDHI

We have taken a cursory view of the different steps in Rāja-yoga except the finer ones, the training in concentration, which is the goal to which Rāja-yoga will lead us. We see, as human beings, that all our knowledge which is called rational is referred to consciousness. My consciousness of this table and of your presence makes me know that the table and you are here. At the same time, there is a very great part of my existence of which I am not conscious: all the different organs inside the body, the different parts of the brain—nobody is conscious of these.

When I eat food I do it consciously; when I assimilate it I do it unconsciously; when the food is manufactured into blood, it is done unconsciously; when out of the blood all the different parts of my body are strengthened, it is done unconsciously. And yet it is I who am doing all this; there cannot be twenty people in this one body. How do I know that I do it, and nobody else? It may be urged that my business is only to eat and assimilate the food, and that the strengthening of the body by the food is done for me by somebody else. That cannot be; because it can be demonstrated that almost every action of which we are now unconscious can be brought up to the plane of consciousness. The heart is beating apparently without our control; none of us can control the heart; it goes on its own way. But by practice men can bring even the heart under control, until it will just beat at will, slowly or quickly, or almost stop. Nearly every part of the body can be brought under control. What does this show? That the functions which are beneath consciousness are also performed by us, only we are performing them unconsciously. We have, then, two planes in which the human mind works. First is the conscious plane, in which all work is always accompanied by the feeling of "I." Next comes the unconscious plane, where the work is unaccompanied by the feeling of "I." That part of the mind's work which is unaccompanied by egoity is unconscious work, and that part which is accompanied by egoity is conscious work. In the lower animals this unconscious work is called instinct. In higher animals, and in the highest of all animals, man, what is called conscious work prevails.

But the matter does not end here. There is a still higher plane on which the mind can work. It can go beyond consciousness. Just as unconscious work is beneath consciousness, so there is another sort of work which is above consciousness and which also is not accompanied by egoity. The feeling of "I" is only on the middle plane. When the mind is above or below that plane, there is no feeling of "I," and yet the mind works. When the mind goes beyond the plane of self-consciousness, it experiences samādhi, or superconsciousness. But how do we know that a man in samādhi has not gone below consciousness, has not degenerated instead of going higher? In both cases the experience is unaccompanied by the feeling of "I." The answer is that by the effects, by the results of the work, we know which is below and which is above. When a man goes into deep sleep he enters a plane beneath consciousness. His body functions all the time: he breathes, perhaps he moves the body in his sleep, without any accompanying feeling of "I"; he is unconscious, and when he returns from his sleep he is the same man who went into it. The sum total of the knowledge which he had before he went to sleep remains the same; it does not increase at all. No enlightenment comes. But when a man goes into samādhi, if he goes into it a fool, he comes out a sage.

What makes the difference? From one state a man comes out the very same man that went in, and from the other state the man comes out enlightened: a sage, a prophet, a saint—his whole character changed, his life changed, illumined. These are two different effects. Now that being so, the causes must be different. As this illumination with which a man comes back fror samādhi is much higher than can be got from unconsciousness, or much higher than can be got by reasoning in a conscious state, it must therefore be superconsciousness, and so samādhi is called the superconscious state.

This, in short, is the idea of samādhi. What is its application? The application is here. The field of reason, or of the conscious working of the mind, is narrow and limited. There is a little circle within which human reason must move. It cannot go beyond. Every attempt to go beyond is futile. Yet it is beyond this circle of reason that there lies all that humanity holds most dear. All these questions—whether there is an immortal Soul, whether there is a God, whether there is any supreme Intelligence guiding this universe, or not—are beyond the field of reason. Reason can never answer these questions. What does reason say? It says, "I am an agnostic; I do not know either yea or nay." Yet these questions are very important to us. Without a proper answer to them human life will be purposeless.

All our ethical theories, all our moral attitudes, all that is good and great in human nature, have been moulded by answers that have come from beyond the circle. It is very important, therefore, that we should have answers to these questions. If life is only a short play, if the universe is only a "fortuitous combination of atoms," then why should I do good to another? Why should there be mercy, justice, or fellow-feeling? The best thing for men in this world would be to make hay while the sun shines—each man for himself. If there is no hope, why should I love my brother and not cut his throat? If there is nothing beyond, if there is no freedom, but only rigorous, dead law, I should only try to make myself happy here. You will find people saying, nowadays, that they make utility the basis of morality. What is this basis? The procuring of the greatest amount of happiness for the greatest number. Why should I do this? Why should I not procure the greatest unhappiness for the greatest number, if that serves my purpose? How will utilitarians answer this question? How do you know what is right or what is wrong? I am impelled by my desire for happiness; I fulfil it because it is my nature to do so; I know nothing beyond. I have these desires and must fulfil them. Why should you complain? Whence come all these truths about human life, about morality, about the immortal Soul, about God, about love and sympathy, about being good, and above all, about being unselfish?

All ethics, all human action, and all human thought hang upon this one idea of unselfishness; the whole ideal of human life can be put into that one word *unselfishness*. Why should we be unselfish? Where is the necessity, the force, the power, that compels me to be unselfish? You call yourself a rational man, a utilitarian, but if you do not show me a reason for your utility, I say you are irrational. Show me the reason why I should not be selfish. To ask one to be unselfish may be good as poetry; but poetry is not the reason. Show me the reason: Why should I be unselfish, and why good? Because Mr. and Mrs. So-and-so say this does not weigh with me. Where is the utility in my being unselfish? If utility means the greatest amount of happiness, for me utility means to be selfish. What is the answer? The utilitarian can never give it. Where did those who preached unselfishness and taught it to the human race get this idea from? We know it is not instinctive; the animals, which act through instinct, do not know it. Neither has it come from reason; reason does not know much about such ideas. Whence, then, did they come?

We find, in studying history, that one fact is held in common by all the great teachers of religion the world has ever had: they all claim to have got their truths from beyond; only many of them did not know where they got them from. For instance, one says that an angel came down, in the form of a human being with wings, and said to him: "Hear, O man! This is the message." Another says that a deva, a bright being, appeared to him. A third says that he dreamt that his ancestor came and told him certain things; he did not know anything beyond that. But this is common: all claim that this knowledge has come to them from beyond, not through their reasoning power. What does the science of Yoga teach? It teaches that they were right in claiming that all this knowledge came to them from beyond reasoning, but also that it came from within themselves.

The yogi teaches that the mind itself has a higher state of existence, beyond reason, a superconscious state, and that when the mind rises to that state, then this knowledge, which is beyond reason, comes— metaphysical and transcendental knowledge comes to that man. This state of going beyond reason, beyond ordinary human knowledge, may sometimes come by chance to a man who does not understand its science; he stumbles upon it, as it were. When he stumbles upon it, he generally interprets it as coming from outside. So this explains why an inspiration, or transcendental knowledge, may be the same in different countries, but in one country it will seem to come through an angel, and in another through a deva, and in a third through God. What does it mean? It means that the mind brought out the knowledge from within itself and that the manner of finding it was interpreted according to the beliefs and education of the person through whom it came. The real fact is that these various men stumbled, as it were, upon this superconscious state.

The yogi says that there is a great danger in stumbling upon this state. In a good many cases there is the danger of the brain's being deranged; and as a rule you will find that all those men, however great they were, who stumbled upon this superconscious state without understanding it groped in the dark and generally had, along with their knowledge, some quaint superstitions. They opened themselves to hallucinations. Mohammed claimed that the Angel Gabriel came to him in a cave one day and took him on the heavenly horse Harak to visit the heavens. But with all that, Mohammed spoke some wonderful truths. If you read the Koran, you find the most wonderful truths mixed with superstitions. How will you explain it? The man was inspired, no doubt, but that inspiration was, as it were, stumbled upon. He was not a trained yogi and did not know the reason for what he was doing. Think of the good Mohammed did to the world, and think of the great evil that has been done through his fanaticism! Think of the millions massacred through his teachings—mothers bereft of their children, children made orphans, whole countries destroyed, millions upon millions of people killed!

So we see this danger when we study the life of a great teacher like Mohammed: Whenever a prophet got into the superconscious state by heightening his emotional nature, he brought away from it not only some truths but some fanaticism also, some superstition which injured the world as much as the greatness of the teaching helped it. Yet we find, at the same time, that all the great teachers were inspired. To get any meaning out of the mass of incongruity we call human life, we have to transcend our reason; but we must do it scientifically, slowly, by regular practice, and we must cast off all superstition. We must take up the study of the superconscious state just like any other science. On reason we must lay our foundation. We must follow reason as far as it leads, and when reason fails, reason itself will show us the way to the highest plane. When you hear a man say, "I am inspired," and then talk irrationally, reject him. Why? Because these three states—instinct, reason, and superconsciousness, or the unconscious, conscious, and superconscious—belong to one and the same mind. There are not three minds in one man, but one state of the mind develops into the others. Instinct develops into reason, and reason into the transcendental consciousness; therefore not one of the states contradicts the others. Real inspiration never contradicts reason, but fulfils it. Just as the great prophets "come not to destroy but to fulfil," so inspiration always comes to fulfil reason and is in harmony with it.

All the different steps in yoga are intended to bring us scientifically to the superconscious state, or samādhi. Furthermore, this is a most vital point to understand: Inspiration is as much in every man's nature as it was in that of the ancient prophets. These prophets were not unique; they were men such as you or I. They were great yogis. They had gained this superconsciousness, and you and I also can gain the same. They were not peculiar people. The very fact that one man ever reached that state proves that it is possible for every man to do so. Not only is it possible, but every man must eventually reach that state—and that is religion. Experience is the only teacher we have. We may talk and reason all our lives, but we shall not understand a word of truth until we experience it ourselves. You cannot hope to make a man a surgeon by simply giving him a few books. You cannot satisfy my curiosity to see a country by showing me a map; I must have actual experience. Maps can only create curiosity in us to get more perfect knowledge. Beyond that, they have no value whatever. Clinging to books only degenerates the human mind. Was there ever a more horrible blasphemy than the statement that all the knowledge of God is confined to this or that book? How dare men call God infinite and yet try to compress Him within the covers of a little book! Millions of people have been killed because they did not believe what the books said, because they would not see all the knowledge of God within the covers of a book. Of course, all this killing and murdering has gone by; but the world is still tremendously bound up in a belief in books.

In order to reach the superconscious state in a scientific manner, it is necessary to pass through the various steps of Rāja-yoga I have been teaching. After pratyāhāra and dhāranā, we come to dhyāna, meditation. When the mind has been trained to remain fixed on a certain internal or external object, there comes to it the power of flowing in an unbroken current, as it were, towards that object. This state is called dhyāna. When one has so intensified the power of dhyāna as to be able to reject the external part of the perception and meditate only on the internal part, the meaning, that state is called samādhi. The three—

dhāranā, dhyāna, and samādhi—together are called samyama. To explain: If the mind can first concentrate upon an object, and then is able to continue in that concentration for a length of time, and then, by continued concentration, can dwell only on the internal part of the perception, of which the object was the effect, or gross part, everything comes under its control.

This meditative state is the highest state of existence. So long as there is desire no real happiness can come. It is only the contemplative, witness-like study of objects that brings us real enjoyment and happiness. The animal has its happiness in the senses, man in his intellect, and the god in spiritual contemplation. It is only to the soul that has attained this contemplative state that the world really becomes beautiful. To him who desires nothing and does not mix himself up with the world the manifold changes of nature are one panorama of beauty and sublimity.

These ideas have to be understood in studying dhyāna, or meditation. We hear a sound. First there is the external vibration; second, the nerve motion that carries it to the mind; third, the reaction from the mind, along with which flashes the knowledge of the object which was the external cause of these different changes, from the ethereal vibrations to the mental reaction. These three are called, in yoga, sabda (sound), artha (meaning), and jnāna (knowledge). In the language of physiology they are called the ethereal vibration, the motion in the nerve and brain, and the mental reaction. Now these, though distinct processes, have become mixed up in such a fashion as to become quite indistinguishable. In fact, we cannot now perceive any of these; we perceive only their combined effect, what we call the external object. Every act of perception includes these three, and there is no reason why we should not be able to distinguish them.

When, by the previous preparations, the mind has become strong and controlled, and gained the power of finer perception, it should be employed in meditation. This meditation must begin with gross objects and slowly rise to finer, until it becomes objectless. The mind should first be employed in perceiving the external causes of sensations, then the internal motions, and then its own reaction. When it has succeeded in perceiving the external causes of sensations by themselves, the mind will acquire the power of perceiving all fine material existences, all fine bodies and forms. When it thus succeeds in perceiving the motions inside by themselves, it will gain the control of all mental waves, in itself or in others, even before they have translated themselves into physical energy. And when the yogi's mind is able to perceive the mental reaction by itself, it will acquire the knowledge of everything, since every sensible object and every thought is the result of this reaction. Then the yogi will have seen the very foundations of his mind, and it will be under his perfect control. Different powers will come to the yogi; if he yields to the temptations of any one of these the road to his farther progress will be barred—such is the evil of running after enjoyments. But if he is strong enough to reject even these miraculous powers, he will attain to the goal of yoga, the complete suppression of the waves in the ocean of the mind. Then the glory of the Soul, undisturbed by distractions of the mind or motions of the body, will shine in its full effulgence, and the yogi will find himself, as he is and as he always was, the Essence of Knowledge, the Immortal, the All-pervading.

Samādhi is the property of every human being—nay, of every animal. From the lowest animal to the highest angel, some time or other each one will have to come to that state; and then, and then alone, will real religion begin for him. Until then we only struggle towards that stage. There is no difference now between us and those who have no religion, because we have no experience. What is concentration good for, save to bring us to this experience? Each one of the steps to attain samādhi has been reasoned out, properly adjusted, and scientifically organized. When faithfully practised, they will surely lead to the desired end. Then will all sorrows cease, all miseries vanish. The seeds of action will be burnt, and the Soul will be free for ever.

RĀJA-YOGA IN BRIEF

THE FOLLOWING is a summary of Rāja-yoga freely translated from the *Kurma Purāna:*

The fire of yoga burns the cage of sin which imprisons a man. Knowledge becomes purified and Nirvāna is directly obtained. From yoga comes knowledge; knowledge, again, helps the yogi to obtain freedom. He who combines in himself both yoga and knowledge—with him the Lord is pleased. Those who practise mahā-yoga either once a day, or twice, or thrice, or always—know them to be gods. Yoga is divided into two parts: one is called abhāva-yoga, and the other, mahā-yoga. That in which one's self is meditated upon as a void and without qualities is called abhāva-yoga. That in which one sees one's self as blissful, bereft of all impurities, and as one with God is called mahā-yoga. The yogi, by either of these, realizes the Self. The other yogas that we read and hear of do not deserve to be ranked with mahā-yoga, in which the yogi finds himself and the whole universe to be God. This is the highest of all yogas.

Yama, niyama, āsana, prānāyāma, pratyāhāra, dhāranā, dhyāna, and samādhi are the steps in Rāja-yoga. Non-injury, truthfulness, non-covetousness, chastity, and not receiving anything from another are called yama, which purifies the mind, the chitta. Never producing pain in any living being, by thought, word, or deed, is what is called ahimsā, non-injury. There is no virtue higher than non-injury. There is no happiness higher than what a man obtains by this attitude of non-offensiveness to all creation. By truthfulness we attain the fruits of work. Through truth everything is attained; in truth everything is established. Relating facts as they are—this is truthfulness. Not taking others' goods by stealth or by force is called asteyam, non-covetousness. Chastity in thought, word, and deed, always and in all conditions, is what is called brahmacharya. Not receiving any present from anybody, even when one is suffering terribly, is what is called aparigraha. The idea is that when a man receives a gift from another, his heart becomes impure, he becomes low, he loses his independence, he becomes bound and attached.

The following are helps to success in yoga and are called niyama, or regular habits and observances: tapas (austerity), svādhyāya (study), santosha (contentment), śaucham (purity), and Iśvara-pranidhāna (worshipping God). Fasting or in other ways controlling the body is called physical tapas. Repeating the Vedas and other mantras, by which the sattva material in the body is purified, is called study, svādhyāya. There are three sorts of repetitions of these mantras. One is called verbal, another semi-verbal, and the third mental. The verbal or audible is the lowest, and the inaudible is the highest of all. Repetition which is loud is the verbal; in the next one only the lips move, but no sound is heard. The inaudible repetition of the mantra, accompanied by the thinking of its meaning, is called mental repetition and is the highest. The sages have said that there are two sorts of purification: external and internal. The purification of the body by water, earth, or other materials is the external purification; bathing is an example. Purification of the mind by truthfulness, and by the other virtues, is what is called the internal purification. Both are necessary for the practice of yoga. It is not enough for a man to be internally pure. When only one is attainable, the internal purity is to be preferred; but no one will be a yogi until he has both. God is worshipped by praise, by thought, and by devotion.

We have spoken about yama and niyama. The next is āsana, posture. The only thing to understand about it is to leave the body free, holding the chest, shoulders, and head straight. Then comes prāṇāyāma. *Prāna* means the vital force in one's own body, and the word *āyāma* means control. There are three sorts of prāṇā-yāma: the very simple, the middle, and the very high. It is further divided into three parts: filling, restraining, and emptying. When you begin with twelve seconds it is the lowest prāṇāyāma; when you begin with twenty-four seconds it is the middle prāṇāyāma; the prāṇāyāma which begins with thirty-six seconds is the best. In the lowest kind of prāṇāyāma there is perspiration; in the medium kind, quivering of the body; and in the highest prāṇāyāma, levitation of the body and influx of great bliss. There is a mantra called the Gāyatri, a very holy verse of the Vedas. It reads: "We meditate on the glory of that Being who has produced this universe; may He enlighten our minds." Om is joined to it at the beginning and the end. In one prāṇāyāma repeat three Gāyatris. All the books speak of prānāyāma's being divided into rechaka (rejecting or exhaling), puraka (inhaling), and kumbhaka (restraining or stationary).

The indriyas, the organs of the senses, are turned outward and come in contact with external objects. Bringing them under the control of the will is what is called pratyāhāra, or gathering towards oneself.

Fixing the mind on the lotus of the heart or on the centre in the head is what is called dhāranā. Confined to one spot as the base, certain mental waves arise; these waves, not swallowed up by other kinds of waves, by degrees become prominent, while the latter recede and finally disappear. Next the multiplicity of the original waves gives place to unity and one wave only is left in the mind. This is dhyāna, meditation.

When no basis is necessary, when the whole of the mind has become one wave, has attained one-formedness, it is called samādhi. Bereft of all association with places and centres, only the meaning of the wave is present. If the mind can be fixed on a centre for twelve seconds it will be a dhāranā; twelve such dhāranās will be a dhyāna; and twelve such dhyānas will be a samādhi.

Where there is apprehension of fire or water, where the ground is strewn with dry leaves, where there are many ant-hills, where there is danger from wild animals, where four streets meet, where there is too much noise, where there are many wicked persons—there yoga must not be practised. This applies more particularly to India. Do not practise when the body feels very lazy or ill, or when the mind is very miserable and sorrowful. Go to a place which is well hidden

and where people do not come to disturb you. Do
not choose dirty places. Rather choose beautiful scenery
or a room in your own house which is beautiful. When
you practise, first salute all the ancient yogis and your
own guru and God, and then begin.

Dhyāna having been explained, a few examples are
given of what to meditate upon. Sit straight and look
at the tip of your nose. Later on we shall come to
know how that helps to concentrate the mind, how by
controlling the two optic nerves one advances a long
way towards the control of the arc of reaction, and so
to the control of the will. Here is one specimen of
meditation: Imagine a lotus upon the top of the head,
several inches up, with virtue as its centre and knowledge as its stalk. The eight petals of the lotus are the
eight powers of the yogi. Inside, the stamens and
pistils are renunciation. If the yogi refuses the external
powers he will come to salvation. So the eight petals of
the lotus are the eight powers, but the internal
stamens and pistils are extreme renunciation, the
renunciation of all these powers. Inside that lotus,
think of the Golden One, the Almighty, the Intangible, whose name is Om, the Inexpressible, surrounded with effulgent light. Meditate on that. An
other meditation is given: Think of a space in your
heart, and think that in the midst of that space a
flame is burning. Think of that flame as your own
soul. Inside the flame is another effulgent light, and
that is the Soul of your soul, God. Meditate upon
that in the heart.

Chastity, non-injury, forgiving even the greatest
enemy, truthfulness, and faith in the Lord—these are

all different vows. Be not afraid if you are not perfect
in all of these. Work and you will succeed. He who
has given up all attachment, all fear, and all anger,
he whose whole soul has gone unto the Lord, he who
has taken refuge in the Lord, whose heart has become
purified—with whatsoever desire he comes to the Lord,
He will grant that to him. Therefore worship Him
through knowledge, love, and renunciation.

"He who hates none, who is the friend of all, who
is merciful to all, who has nothing of his own, who
is free from egotism, who is even-minded in pain and
pleasure, who is forbearing, who is always satisfied,
who is ever devoted to yoga, whose self has become
controlled, whose will is firm, whose mind and intellect are given unto Me—such a one is My beloved
bhakta. He from whom comes no disturbance, who
cannot be disturbed by others, who is free from joy,
fear, and anxiety—such a one is My beloved. He
who does not depend on anything, who is pure and
active, who does not care whether good comes or evil,
and never becomes miserable, who has given up all
efforts for himself, who is the same in praise or in
blame, silent and thoughtful, pleased with what little
comes his way, homeless, having the whole world for
his home, and steady in his mind—such a one is My
beloved bhakta."[1] Such a one becomes a yogi.

*   *   *

There was a great god-sage called Nārada. Just as
there are sages among men, great yogis, so there are
great yogis among the gods. Nārada was a great yogi,
and renowned. He travelled everywhere. One day he

[1] Bhagavad Gītā XII. 13-20.

was passing through a forest and saw a man who had been meditating until the white ants had built a huge mound around his body—he had been sitting in that position so long. He said to Nārada, "Where are you going?" Nārada replied, "I am going to heaven." "Then ask God when He will be merciful to me, when I shall attain freedom." Farther on Nārada saw another man. He was jumping about, singing and dancing, and said, "O Nārada, where are you going?" His voice and his gestures were wild. Nārada said, "I am going to heaven." "Then ask when I shall be free." Nārada went on. In the course of time he came again by the same road, and there was the man who had been meditating with the ant-hill around him. He said, "O Nārada, did you ask the Lord about me?" "Oh, yes." "What did He say?" "The Lord told me that you would attain freedom in four more births." Then the man began to weep and wail, and said, "I have meditated until an ant-hill has grown around me, and I have yet four more births!" Nārada went to the other man. "Did you ask my question?" "Oh, yes. Do you see this tamarind tree? I have to tell you that you shall be born as many times as there are leaves on that tree, and then you shall attain freedom." The man began to dance for joy, and said, "Ah, I shall have freedom after such a short time!" A voice came, "My child, you will have freedom this minute." That was the reward for his perseverance. He was ready to work through all those births; nothing discouraged him. But the first man felt that even four more births were too long. Only perseverance like that of the man who was willing to wait aeons brings about the highest result.

INTRODUCTION TO
PATANJALI'S YOGA APHORISMS

B EFORE GOING INTO the *Yoga Aphorisms* I shall try
to discuss one great question, upon which, for the
yogis, rests the whole theory of religion. It seems to be
the consensus of opinion of the great minds of the
world, and it has been nearly demonstrated by researches into physical nature, that we are the outcome
and manifestation of an absolute condition, which lies
behind our present relative condition, and that we
shall return to that absolute condition. This being
granted, the question is, which is better, the absolute
state or this present state? There are not wanting
people who think that the manifested state is the
higher state of man. Thinkers of great calibre are of
the opinion that we are manifestations of undiffer-
entiated being, and that the differentiated state is
higher than the absolute. They imagine that in the
absolute state there cannot be any quality; that it must
be insensate, dull, and lifeless; that only this life can
be enjoyed, and therefore we must cling to it.

First of all let us inquire into other solutions of life.
There was an old solution that man remained the
same after death, that all his good qualities, minus his
evil ones, remained for ever. Logically stated, this
means that man's goal is the world; this world carried
a stage higher, and purified of its evils, is the state
94

called heaven. The theory, on the face of it, is absurd and puerile, because such a state cannot exist. There cannot be good without evil, or evil without good. A world where there is all good and no evil is what Indian logicians call a "castle in the air."

Another theory in modern times has been presented by several schools: that man's destiny is to go on always improving, always struggling towards, but never reaching, the goal. This statement, though apparently very nice, is also absurd, because there is no such thing as motion in a straight line. Every motion is in a circle. If you take up a stone and throw it into space, and then live long enough, that stone, if it meets with no obstruction, will come back exactly to your hand. A straight line, infinitely projected, must end in a circle. Therefore this idea that the destiny of man is to progress ever forward and forward, without ever stopping, is absurd. Although it is extraneous to the subject, I may remark that the idea of motion's being in a circle explains the ethical theory that you must not hate, but must love. Just as, according to the modern theory, the electric current leaves the dynamo, completes the circle, and comes back to the dynamo, so also hate and love: they must come back to the source. Therefore do not hate anybody, because that hatred which goes out from you must in the long run come back to you. If you love, that love will come back to you, completing the circle. It is as certain as can be that every bit of hatred that goes out of the heart of a man comes back to him in full force; nothing can stop it. Similarly every impulse of love comes back to him.

On other and more practical grounds we see that
the theory of eternal progression is untenable; for
destruction is the end of everything earthly. All our
struggles and hopes and fears and joys—what will
they lead to? We shall all end in death. Nothing is so
certain as this. Where, then, is this motion in a
straight line, this infinite progression? It only means
going out to a distance and coming back to the centre
from which one started. See how from nebulae the
sun, moon, and stars are produced, and then dissolve
and go back to nebulae. The same is happening
everywhere. The plant takes its substance from the
earth, decays, and gives it back to the earth. Every
form in this world is taken out of surrounding atoms
and goes back to these atoms. It cannot be that the
same law acts differently in different places. Law is
uniform; nothing is more certain than that. If this is
the law of nature, it also applies to the mind. The
mind will dissolve and go back to its origin. Whether
we will or no, we shall have to return to our origin,
which is called God, or the Absolute. We have all
come from God and we are all bound to go back to
God; call it by any name you like—God, the Absolute, or nature—the fact remains the same. "From
whom all this universe comes out, in whom all that is
born lives, and to whom all returns." This is one fact
that is certain. Nature works on the same plan; what
is being worked out in one sphere is repeated in
millions of spheres. What you see in the planets, the
same will be with this earth, with men, and with all.
The huge wave consists of small waves—it may be of
millions of them. Likewise, the life of the whole world

is compounded of the lives of millions of little beings, and the death of the whole world is compounded of the deaths of these millions of little beings.

Now the question arises, is going back to God the higher state, or not? The philosophers of the Yoga school emphatically answer that it is. They say that man's present state is a degeneration; there is not one religion on the face of the earth which says that man is an improvement. The idea is that his beginning is perfect and pure, then he degenerates until he cannot degenerate further, and finally there must come a time when he shoots upward again to complete the circle; the circle must be described. However low he may go, he must ultimately take the upward curve and go back to the original source, which is God. Man comes from God in the beginning, in the middle he becomes man, and in the end he goes back to God. This is the way of putting it in the dualistic form. The monistic form is that man *is* God and becomes God again. If our present state is the higher one, then why is there so much horror and misery, and why is there an end to it? If this is the higher state, why does it end? That which corrupts and degenerates cannot be the highest state. Why should it be so diabolical, so unsatisfying? It is only excusable inasmuch as, through it, we are able to reach a higher stage; we have to pass through it in order to become regenerate. Put a seed into the ground and it disintegrates, dissolves, after a time; and out of that dissolution comes a splendid tree. Every soul must disintegrate in order that it may become God. So it follows that the sooner we get out of this state we call manhood, the better

for us. Is it by committing suicide that we get out of
this state? Not at all. That would be making it worse.
Torturing ourselves or condemning the world is not
the way to get out. We have to pass through the
Slough of Despond, and the sooner we are through,
the better. It must always be remembered that manhood is not the highest state.

The really difficult part to understand is that the
Absolute, which has been called the highest state, is
not, as some fear, that of the zoophyte or the stone.
According to them there are only two states of
existence: one, that of the stone, and the other, that
of thought. What right have they to limit existence
to these two? Is there not something infinitely superior
to thought? The vibrations of light, when they are
very low, we do not see. When they become a little
more intense they become light to us. When they
become still more intense we do not see them; it is
dark to us. Is the darkness in the end the same darkness as that in the beginning? Certainly not; they are
different as the poles. Is the absence of thought in
the stone the same as the absence of thought in God?
Certainly not. God does not think; He does not reason.
Why should He? Is anything unknown to Him, that
He should reason? The stone *cannot* reason; God *does*
not. That is the difference. These philosophers think
it is awful if we go beyond thought; they find nothing
beyond thought. But there is a much higher state of
existence than reasoning. It is really beyond the intellect that the first state of religious life is to be found.
When you step beyond thought and intellect and all
reasoning, then you have made the first step towards

God; and that is the beginning of life. What is commonly called life is but an embryo state.

The next question will be: What proof is there that the state beyond thought and reasoning is the highest state? In the first place, all the great men of the world, much greater than those who only talk—men who move the world, men who never think of any selfish ends whatever—declare that this life is but a little stage on the way towards Infinity, which is beyond. In the second place, they not only say so, but show the way to everyone, explain their methods, that all may follow in their steps. In the third place, there is no other way left. There is no other explanation. Taking it for granted that there is no higher state, why are we going through this circle all the time? What can explain the world's existence? If we cannot go farther, if we must not ask for anything more, our knowledge will be limited to the sensible world. This is what is called agnosticism. But what reason is there to believe the testimony of the senses? I would call that man a true agnostic who would stand still in the street and die. If reason is all in all, then we must accept nihilism and shall have no place to stand. If a man is agnostic about everything but money, fame, and name, he is only a fraud. Immanuel Kant has said, no doubt, that we cannot penetrate beyond the tremendous dead wall called reason. But that we *can* go beyond reason is the very first idea upon which all Indian thought takes its stand; it dares to seek, and succeeds in finding, something higher than reason, where alone the explanation of the present state is to be found. This is the value of the study of Yoga, which will take us beyond reason. "Thou art our Father, who takest us to the other shore of this ocean of ignorance." This going beyond ignorance, and nothing else, is the goal of religion.

CONCENTRATION: ITS SPIRITUAL USES

1

Now yoga is explained.

2

Yoga is the restraining of the mind-stuff (chitta) from taking various forms (vrittis).

A good deal of explanation is necessary here. We have to understand what the chitta is and what the vrittis are. I have eyes. The eyes do not really see. Take away the nerve centre which is in the brain; the eyes will still be there, with the retinae complete, as also the pictures of objects on them, and yet the eyes will not see. So the eyes are only a secondary instrument, not the organ of vision. The organ of vision is in a nerve centre in the brain. The two eyes will not be sufficient. Sometimes a man is asleep with his eyes open. The light is there and the picture is there, but a third thing is necessary: the mind must be joined to the organ. So the eye is merely the external instrument; we need also the centre in the brain and the agency of the mind. Carriages roll down a street and you do not hear them. Why? Because your mind has not attached itself to the organ of hearing. First there is the instrument, second, the organ, and third, the mind's attachment to these two. The mind takes the impression farther in and presents it to the determina-

101

tive faculty, or buddhi, which reacts. Along with this reaction flashes the idea of ego. Then this mixture of action and reaction is presented to the Purusha, the real Soul, which perceives an object in this mixture.

The organs (indriyas), the mind (manas), the determinative faculty (buddhi), and egoity (ahamkāra) —all these together form the group called the antahkarana, the internal instrument. They are but various processes in the mind-stuff, or chitta. The waves of thought in the chitta are called vrittis (literally, whirlpools).

What is thought? Thought is a force, as is gravitation or repulsion. From the infinite storehouse of force in nature, the instrument called the chitta takes hold of some, absorbs it, and sends it out as thought. Force is supplied to us through food, and out of that food the body obtains the power of motion, and so forth. Others, the finer forces, it sends out as what we call thought. So we see that the mind is not intelligent; yet it appears to be intelligent. Why so? Because the intelligent Soul is behind it. The Soul is the only sentient being; the mind is merely the instrument through which It perceives the external world. Take this book: as a book it does not exist outside; what exists outside is unknown and unknowable. The unknowable furnishes the suggestion that gives a blow to the mind, and the mind gives out the reaction in the form of a book, just as when a stone is thrown into the water, the water is thrown against it in the form of waves. The real universe is the occasion of the reaction of the mind. A book form or an elephant form or a man form is not outside; all that we know is our mental reaction from the outer suggestion. "Matter is the permanent possibility of sensations," said John Stuart Mill. It is only the suggestion that is outside. Take an oyster for example. You know how pearls are made. A parasite gets inside the shell and causes irritation, and the oyster throws a sort of enamelling round it, and this makes the pearl. The universe of experience is our own enamel, so to say, and the real universe is the parasite serving as nucleus. The ordinary man will never understand it, because when he tries to do so, he throws out an enamel and sees only his own enamel.

Now we understand what is meant by these vrittis. The real man is behind the mind; the mind is the instrument in his hands. It is his intelligence that is percolating through the mind. It is only when you stand behind the mind that it becomes intelligent. When you give it up it falls to pieces and becomes nothing. Thus you understand what is meant by the chitta. It is the mind-stuff, and the vrittis are the waves and ripples rising in it when external causes impinge on it. These vrittis are our universe.

The bottom of a lake we cannot see, because its surface is covered with ripples. It is only possible for us to catch a glimpse of the bottom when the ripples have subsided and the water is calm. If the water is muddy, or is agitated all the time, the bottom will not be seen. If it is clear and there are no waves, we shall see the bottom. The bottom of the lake is our own true Self; the lake is the chitta, and the waves are the vrittis. Again, the mind has three states, one of which is darkness, called tamas, found in brutes and idiots; it only acts to injure. No other idea comes into that state of mind. Then there is the active state of mind, rajas, whose chief motives are power and enjoyment: "I will be powerful and rule others." Then there is the state called sattva, serenity, calmness, in which the waves cease and the water of the mind-lake becomes clear. It is not inactive; rather, it is intensely active. It is the greatest manifestation of power to be calm. It is easy to be active. Let the reins go and the horses will run away with you. Anyone can do that; but he who can stop the plunging horses is the strong man. Which requires the greater strength, letting go or restraining? The calm man is not the man who is dull. You must not mistake sattva for dullness or laziness. The calm man is the one who has control over the mind's waves. Activity is the manifestation of inferior strength; calmness, of superior.

The chitta is always trying to get back to its natural pure state, but the organs draw it out. To restrain it, to check this outward tendency, and to start it on the return journey to the Essence of Intelligence is the first step in yoga, because only in this way can the chitta get into its proper state.

Although the chitta exists in every animal, from the lowest to the highest, it is only in the human being that we find it as the intellect. Until the mind-stuff can take the form of intellect, it is not possible for it to return through all these steps and liberate the soul. Immediate salvation is impossible for the cow or the dog, although they have minds, because their chitta cannot as yet take that form which we call intellect.

The chitta manifests itself in the following forms:

scattering, darkening, gathering, one-pointed, and con-centrated. The "scattering" form is activity. Its tend-ency is to manifest itself in the form of pleasure or of pain. The "darkening" form is dullness, which tends to injury. The commentator says that the first form is natural to the devas, the gods, and the second to the demons. The "gathering" form functions when the chitta struggles to draw itself to its centre; the "one-pointed" form, when it tries to concentrate. And the "concentrated" form brings us to samādhi.

3

At that time (i.e. the time of concentration) the Seer (Purusha) rests in His own [unmodified] state.

As soon as the waves have stopped and the lake has become quiet, we see its bottom. So with the mind: when it is calm, we see what our own nature is; we do not mix ourselves with the modifications of the mind, but remain our own selves.

4

At other times (i.e. when not concentrating) the Seer is identified with the modifications.

For instance, someone blames me; this produces a modification, vritti, in my mind, and I identify myself with it, and the result is misery.

5

There are five classes of modifications, [some] painful and [others] not painful.

6

[These are] right knowledge, indiscrimination, verbal delusion, sleep, and memory.

7

Direct perception, inference, and competent evidence constitute right knowledge, or proof.

When two of our perceptions do not contradict each other we call it a proof. I hear something, and if it contradicts something already perceived, I do not believe it and begin to fight it out. There are three kinds of proof. Direct perception, pratyaksha, whatever we see and feel, is its own proof, if there has been nothing to delude the senses. I see the world; that is sufficient proof that it exists. Secondly, anumāna, inference: you see a sign, and from the sign you come to the thing signified. Thirdly, āptavākya, the direct perception of the yogis, of those who have seen Truth. We are all of us struggling towards knowledge. You and I have to struggle hard and come to knowledge through a long, tedious process of reasoning; but the yogi, the pure one, has gone beyond all this. To him the past, the present, and the future alike are one book for his mind to read; he does not have to go through the tedious processes for obtaining knowledge that we have to; his words are their own proof, because he sees knowledge in himself. These, for instance, are the authors of the sacred scriptures; therefore the scriptures are their own proof. If any such persons are living now their words will be their own proof. Other philosophers go into long discussions about āptavākya and they ask, "What is the proof of their words?" The proof is their direct perception. Because whatever I see is its own proof, and whatever you see is its own proof, if it does not contradict any past knowledge. There is knowledge beyond the senses, and whenever it does not contradict reason and past human experience, that knowledge is its own proof. Any madman may come into this room and say that he sees angels around him; that would not be sufficient proof. In the first place, it must be true knowledge, and secondly, it must not contradict past knowledge, and thirdly, it must depend upon the character of the man who gives it out. I hear it said that the character of the man is not of so much importance as what he may say; we must first hear what he says. This may be true in other things: a man may be wicked and yet make an astronomical discovery; but in religion it is different, because no impure man will ever have the power to preach the truths of religion.

Therefore we have first of all to see that the man who declares himself to be an āpta is a perfectly unselfish and holy person; secondly, that he has gone beyond the senses; and thirdly, that what he says does not contradict the past knowledge of humanity. Any new discovery of truth must not contradict past truth, but must fit into it. And fourthly, we have to see that that truth has a possibility of verification. If a man says, "I have seen a vision," and tells me that I cannot see it, I will not believe him. Everyone must have the power to see it for himself. Further, no one who sells his knowledge is an āpta. All these conditions must be fulfilled: You must first see that the man is pure and that he has no selfish motive, that he has no thirst for gain or fame; secondly, he must show that he has had superconscious experience; thirdly, he must give us something which we cannot get from our

senses and which is for the benefit of the world. And
we must see that it does not contradict other truths;
if it contradicts them we must reject it at once.
Fourthly, the man should never be an exception; he
should represent only what all men can attain. The
three sorts of proof are, then, direct sense perception,
inference, and the words of an āpta. I cannot trans-
late this word into English. It is not "one who is inspired," because inspiration is believed to come from
outside, while this knowledge comes from the man
himself. The literal meaning is "one who has attained."

8

**Indiscrimination is false knowledge not based on
the real nature [of an object].**

The next class of vrittis that arises is the mistaking
of one thing for another, as a piece of mother-of-pearl
is mistaken for a piece of silver.

9

**Verbal delusion follows from words having no
[corresponding] reality.**

There is another class of vrittis called vikalpa. A
word is uttered, and we do not wait to consider its
meaning; we jump to a conclusion immediately. It is a
sign of weakness of the chitta. Now you can understand the importance of restraint. The weaker the
man, the less he has of restraint. Examine yourselves
always by that test. When you are about to become
angry or miserable, reason it out and see how some

news that has come to you is throwing your mind into vrittis.

10

Sleep is a vritti which embraces the feeling of voidness.

The next class of vrittis is called sleep, comprising dream and deep sleep. When we awake we know that we were sleeping; we can only have memory of perception. That which we do not perceive we never can have any memory of. Every reaction is a wave in the lake. Now if, during sleep, the mind had no waves, it would have no perceptions, positive or negative, and therefore we should not remember them. The very reason of our remembering sleep is that during sleep there was a certain class of waves in the mind. Memory is another class of vrittis; it is called smriti.

11

Memory arises when [the vrittis of] perceived objects do not slip away [and through impressions come back to consciousness].

Memory can come from direct perception, false knowledge, verbal delusion, and sleep. For instance, you hear a word. That word is like a stone thrown into the lake of the chitta; it causes a ripple, and that ripple rouses a series of ripples. This is memory. So it is in sleep. When the peculiar kind of ripple called sleep throws the chitta into a ripple of memory, it is called a dream. Dreaming is another form of the ripple which in the waking state is called memory.

12

These [vrittis] are controlled by practice and non-
attachment.

The mind, to have non-attachment, must be clear,
good, and rational. Why should we practise? Because
actions are like the vibrations quivering over the surface of the lake. The vibrations die out, and what is
left? The samskāras, the impressions. When a large
number of these impressions is left on the mind, they
coalesce and become a habit. It is said that habit is
second nature. It is first nature also, and the whole
nature of man; everything that we are is the result
of habit. That gives us consolation; for if it is only
habit, we can make and unmake it at any time. The
samskāras are left by these vibrations, which pass out
of our mind, each one of them leaving its result. Our
character is the sum total of these impressions, and
according as a particular wave prevails one takes that
tone. If good prevails, one becomes good; if wickedness, one becomes wicked; if joyfulness, one becomes
happy. The only remedy for bad habits is counter-
habits; all the bad habits that have left their impressions are to be controlled by good habits. Go on doing
good, thinking holy thoughts, continuously; that is the
only way to suppress base impressions. Never say any
man is hopeless, because he only represents a character, a bundle of habits, which can be checked by
new and better ones. Character is repeated habits, and
repeated habits alone can reform character.

13

Continuous struggle to keep them (the vrittis) perfectly restrained is practice.

What is practice? It is the attempt to keep the mind under restraint, to prevent its going out into waves.

14

It becomes firmly grounded by long and constant efforts with great love [for the end to be attained].

Restraint does not come in a day, but by long continued practice.

15

The subjugation of the thirst for objects seen or heard of is non-attachment.

The motive powers of our actions are two: what we see ourselves, and the experience of others. These two forces throw the mind, the lake, into various waves. Non-attachment is the power of battling against these forces and holding the mind in check. The renunciation of these is what we want. I am passing through a street, and a man comes and takes away my watch. That is my own experience. I see it myself, and it immediately throws my chitta into a wave, taking the form of anger. Do not allow that to come. If you cannot prevent it, you are nothing; if you can, you have vairāgya. Again, the experience of the worldly-minded tells us that sense enjoyments are the highest ideal. These are tremendous temptations. To deny them and not allow the mind to break into waves with regard to them is renunciation; to control the twofold motive powers arising from my own experience and from the experience of others, and thus prevent the chitta from being governed by them, is vairāgya. These should be controlled by me, and not I by them. This sort of mental strength is called renunciation. Vairāgya is the only way to freedom.

16

That is extreme non-attachment which gives up even the thirst for the gunas, and which comes from the knowledge of [the real nature of] the Purusha.

The highest manifestation of the power of vairāgya occurs when it takes away even our attraction towards the gunas. We have first to understand what the Purusha, the Self, is, and what the gunas are. According to the Yoga philosophy the whole of nature consists of three gunas, that is to say, factors or forces; one is called tamas, another rajas, and the third sattva. These three gunas manifest themselves in the physical world as darkness or inactivity, attraction or repulsion, and the equilibrium of the two. Everything that is in nature, all manifestations, are combinations and recombinations of these three forces. Nature has been divided into various categories by the Sāmkhya philosophy; the Self of man is beyond all these, beyond nature. It is effulgent, pure, and perfect. Whatever intelligence we see in nature is but the reflection of this Self upon nature. Nature itself is insentient. You must remember that the word *nature* also includes the mind. Mind is in nature; thought is in nature; from thought down to the grossest form of matter, everything is in nature, is the manifestation of nature. This nature has covered the Self of man, and when nature takes away the covering, the Self appears in Its own glory. Nonattachment, described in aphorism 15 as being the subjugation of the thirst for objects, or nature, is the greatest help towards manifesting the Self. The next aphorism defines samādhi, perfect concentration, which is the goal of the yogi.

17

The samādhi endowed with right knowledge is that which is attended by reasoning, discrimination, bliss, and unqualified ego.

Samādhi is divided into two kinds: one is called samprajnāta, and the other, asamprajnāta. In samprajnāta samādhi come all the powers of controlling nature. It is of four varieties. The first variety is called savitarka, when the mind meditates upon an object again and again, by isolating it from other objects. There are two sorts of objects for meditation in the twenty-five categories of Sāmkhya: the twenty-four insentient categories of nature, and the one sentient Purusha. This part of Yoga is based entirely on Sāmkhya philosophy, about which I have already told you. As you will remember, ego and will and mind have a common basis, the chitta or mind-stuff, out of which they are all manufactured. This mind-stuff takes in the forces of nature and projects them as thought. There must be something, again, where both force and matter are one. This is called avyakta, the unmanifested state of nature before creation, to which, after the end of a cycle, the whole of nature returns, and from which it comes out again at the time of the next creation. Beyond that is the Purusha, the Essence of Intelligence.

Knowledge is power, and as soon as we begin to know a thing we get power over it; so also, when the mind begins to meditate on the different elements it gains power over them. That sort of meditation where the external gross elements are the objects is called savitarka. Vitarka means "question"; savitarka, "with question." This samādhi implies the questioning of the elements, as it were, that they may yield their powers to the man who meditates upon them. There is no liberation in getting powers. It is a search after worldly enjoyments, and there is no real enjoyment in this life. All search for enjoyment is vain; this is the old, old lesson which man finds so hard to learn. When he does learn it, he gets out of the universe and becomes free. The possession of what are called occult powers only intensifies worldliness, and, in the end, intensifies suffering. Though as a scientist Patanjali is bound to point out the possibilities of his science, he never misses an opportunity to warn us against these powers.

Again, in the very same meditation, when one struggles to take the elements out of time and space, and thinks of them as they are, it is called nirvitarka samādhi, "samādhi without question." When the meditation goes a step higher and takes the tanmātras as its object, and thinks of them as within time and space, it is called savichāra samādhi, "samādhi with discrimination"; and when in the same meditation one eliminates time and space and thinks of the fine elements as they are, it is called nirvichāra samādhi, "samādhi without discrimination."

In the next step the elements, both gross and fine, are given up and the object of meditation is the interior organ, the thinking organ. When the thinking organ is thought of as bereft of the qualities of activity and dullness, then follows the sānanda or blissful samādhi. When the mind itself, free from the impurity of rajas and tamas, is the object of meditation, when meditation becomes very ripe and concentrated, when all ideas of the gross and fine materials are given up, when only the sattva state of the ego remains, but differentiated from all other objects, it is called asmitā samādhi. Even in this state one does not completely transcend the mind. The man who has attained it is called in the Vedas videha, or "bereft of body." He can think of himself as without his gross body; but he will have to think of himself as having a fine body. Those who in this state get merged in nature without attaining the goal are called prakritilinas; but those who do not stop even here reach the goal, which is freedom.

18

There is another samādhi, which is attained by constant practice of the cessation of all mental activity, and in which the chitta retains only the unmanifested impressions.

This is the perfect superconscious asamprajnāta samādhi, the state which gives us freedom. The first state does not give us freedom, does not liberate the soul. A man may attain all the powers and yet fall again. There is no safeguard until the soul goes beyond nature. It is very difficult to do so although the method seems easy. The method is to meditate on the mind itself, and whenever any thought comes, to strike it down, allowing no thought to come into the mind, thus making it an entire vacuum. When we can really do this, that very moment we shall attain liberation. When persons without training and preparation try to make their minds vacant, they are likely to succeed only in covering themselves with tamas, the material of ignorance, which makes the mind dull and stupid and leads them to think that they are making a vacuum of the mind. To be able to really do that is to manifest the greatest strength, the highest control.

When this state, asamprajnāta, or superconsciousness, is reached, the samādhi becomes seedless. What is meant by that? In a concentration where there is consciousness, where the mind succeeds only in quelling the waves in the chitta and holding them down, the waves remain in the form of tendencies. These tendencies, or seeds, become waves again when the opportunity comes. But when you have destroyed all these tendencies, almost destroyed the mind, then the samādhi becomes seedless; there are no more seeds in the mind out of which to manufacture again and again this plant of life, this ceaseless round of birth and death.

You may ask what that state would be in which there is no mind, no knowledge. What we call knowledge is a lower state than one beyond knowledge. You must always bear in mind that the extremes look very much alike. If a very low vibration of ether is taken as darkness, and an intermediate state as light, a very high vibration will be darkness again. Similarly, ignorance is the lowest state, knowledge is the middle state, and beyond knowledge is the highest state; the two extremes seem the same. Knowledge itself is a manufactured something, a combination; it is not Reality.

What is the result of constant practice of this higher concentration? All old tendencies of restlessness and dullness will be destroyed, as well as the tendencies of goodness too. The case is similar to that of the chemicals used to take the dross from gold ore. When the ore is smelted, the dross is burnt along with the chemicals. So this constant controlling power will destroy the previous bad tendencies, and eventually the good ones also. Those good and evil tendencies will destroy each other, leaving alone the Soul in Its own splendour, untrammelled by either good or bad, omnipresent, omnipotent, and omniscient. Then the man will know that he had neither birth nor death nor need of heaven or earth. He will know that he neither came nor went; it was nature which was moving, and that movement was reflected upon the Soul. The form of the light reflected by a glass upon the wall moves, and the wall foolishly thinks it is moving. So with all of us: it is the chitta that is constantly moving, making itself into various forms, and we think that we are these various forms. All these delusions will vanish. When that free Soul commands—not prays or begs, but commands—then whatever It desires will be immediately fulfilled; whatever It wants It will be able to do.

According to the Sāmkhya philosophy there is no God. It says that there can be no God of this universe, because if there were one, He must be a soul, and a soul must be either bound or free. How can the soul that is bound by nature, or controlled by nature, create? It is itself a slave. On the other hand, why should the Soul, which is free, create and manipulate all these things? It has no desires; so it cannot have any need to create. Secondly, it says that the theory of God is an unnecessary one; nature explains all. What is the use of any God? But Kapila teaches that there are many souls, who, though nearly attaining perfection, fall short because they cannot completely renounce all powers. Their minds for a time merge in nature, to re-emerge as its masters. These souls are called gods. Such gods there are. We shall all become gods, and according to Sāmkhya, the God spoken of in the Vedas really means one of these free souls. Beyond them there is not an eternally free and blessed Creator of the universe.

On the other hand, the yogis say: "Not so. There is a God; there is one Soul separate from all other souls, and He is the eternal Master of all creation, the Ever Free, the Teacher of all teachers." The yogis admit that those whom Sāmkhya calls the "merged in nature" also exist. They are yogis who have fallen short of perfection; though for a time debarred from attaining the goal, they remain as rulers of parts of the universe.

19

[This samādhi, when not followed by extreme non-attachment,] becomes the cause of the remanifestation of the gods and of those who become merged in nature.

The gods in the Indian systems of philosophy represent certain high offices which are filled successively by various souls. But none of them is perfect.

20

By others [this samādhi] is attained through faith, energy, memory, concentration, and discrimination of the real [from the unreal].

The aphorism refers to those who do not want the position of gods or even that of rulers of cycles; they attain to liberation.

21

Success is speedy for the extremely energetic.

22

The success of yogis differs according as the means they adopt are mild, medium, or intense.

23

Or [this samādhi is attained] by devotion to Iśvara.

24

Iśvara (the Supreme Ruler) is a special Purusha, untouched by misery, actions and their results, and desires.

We must again remember that Patanjali's Yoga philosophy is based upon the Sāmkhya philosophy, the difference being that in the latter there is no place for God, while with the yogis God has a place. The yogis, however, do not associate with God the idea of creating or preserving the universe. God as the Creator of the universe is not what is meant by the Iśvara of the yogis. According to the Vedas, Iśvara is the Creator of the universe; because it is harmonious, it must be the manifestation of one will. The yogis, too, want to establish a God, but they arrive at Him in a peculiar fashion of their own. They say:

25

In Him becomes infinite that all-knowingness which in others is [only] a germ.

The mind always travels between two extremes. You can think of a limited space, but that very idea gives you also unlimited space. Close your eyes and think of a little circle; at the same time that you perceive the little circle, you perceive a circle round it of unlimited dimensions. It is the same with time. Try to think of a second; you will have, with the same act of perception, to think of time which is unlimited. So with knowledge. Knowledge is only a germ in man; but you will have to think of infinite knowledge around it. So the very constitution of our minds shows us that there is unlimited knowledge, and the yogis say that that unlimited knowledge belongs to God.

26

He is the Teacher of even the ancient teachers, not being limited by time.

It is true that all knowledge is within ourselves; but this has to be called forth by another knowledge. Although the capacity to know is within us, this capacity must be awakened. The inner knowledge can be called forth, a yogi maintains, only through another knowledge. Dead, insentient matter can never call forth knowledge; it is the power of knowledge that brings out knowledge. Knowing beings must help us to awaken what is in us; so these teachers are always necessary. The world has never been without them, and no knowledge can be had without them. God is the Teacher of all teachers, because these teachers, however great they may have been—even gods or angels—are all bound and limited by time, while God is not.

There are two peculiar deductions of the yogis. The first is that in thinking of the limited, the mind must also think of the unlimited, and that if one part of that perception is true, so also must the other be, for the reason that their value as perceptions of the mind is equal. The very fact that man has a little knowledge shows that God has unlimited knowledge. If I am to take one, why not the other? Reason forces me to take both or reject both. If I believe that there is a man with a little knowledge, I must also admit that there is Someone behind him with unlimited knowledge. The second deduction is that no knowledge can come without a teacher. It is true, as the modern philosophers say, that there is something in man which evolves out of him. All knowledge is in man; but certain environments are necessary to call it out. We cannot find any knowledge without

teachers. Yet though there are men teachers, god
teachers, and angel teachers, they are all limited. Who
was the teacher before them? We are forced to admit,
finally, one Teacher who is not limited by time; and
that Teacher, of infinite knowledge and without
beginning or end, is called God.

27

The word that manifests Him is Om.

Every thought that you have in the mind has a
counterpart in a word; the word and the thought are
inseparable. The external part of a thing is what we
call word, and the internal part of that same thing
is what we call thought. No man can, by analysis,
separate thought from word. The idea that language
was created by men, certain men sitting together and
deciding upon words, has been proved to be wrong.
So long as man has existed there have been words and
language.

What is the connexion between a thought and a
word? Although we see that there must always be a
word with a thought, it is not necessarily true that
the same thought requires the same word. The thought
may be the same in twenty different countries, yet
the language is different. We must have a word to
express each thought, but these words need not necessarily have the same sound. Sounds will vary in different nations. A commentator says: "Although the
relation between thought and word is perfectly natural,
yet it does not mean a rigid connexion between a
thought and a sound." The sounds vary, yet the relation between the sounds and the thoughts is a natural

one. The connexion between thoughts and sounds is good only if there is a real connexion between the thing signified and the symbol; until then that symbol will never come into general use. The symbol is the manifester of the thing signified, and if the thing signified is already existing, and if, by experience, we know that the symbol has expressed that thing many times, then we are sure that there is a real relation between them. Even if the thing is not present, there will be thousands who will know it by its symbol. There must be a natural connexion between the symbol and the thing signified; then, when that symbol is pronounced, it recalls the thing signified.

Patanjali says that the word that manifests God is Om. Why does he emphasize this word? There are hundreds of words for God. One thought is connected with a great many words; the idea of God is connected with hundreds of words, and each one stands as a symbol for God. Very good. But there must be a generalization among all these words, some substratum, some common ground of all these symbols; and that which is the common symbol will be the best and will really represent them all. In making a sound we use the larynx and the palate as a sounding-board. Is there any articulate sound of which all other sounds are manifestations, one which is the most natural sound? Om (Aum) is such a sound, the basis of all sounds. The first letter, A,[1] is the root sound, the key, pronounced without touching any part of the tongue or palate; M represents the last sound in the series, being produced with closed lips, and the U rolls from

[1] Pronounced like *aw* in *dawn*.

the very root to the end of the sounding-board of the mouth. Thus Om represents the whole phenomenon of sound-production. As such, it must be the natural symbol, the matrix of all the various sounds. It denotes the whole range and possibility of all the words that can be uttered.

Apart from these speculations, we see that around this word *Om* are centred all the different religious ideas in India; all the various religious ideas of the Vedas have gathered themselves around this word. What has that to do with America and England, or any other country? Simply this: that the word has been retained at every stage of religious growth in India and has been manipulated to mean all the various ideas about God. Monists, dualists, mono-dualists, separatists, and even atheists have taken up this Om. Om has become the one symbol for the religious aspiration of the vast majority of human beings. Take, for instance, the English word *God*. It covers only a limited function; and if you go beyond it you have to add adjectives to make it the Personal or Impersonal or Absolute God. So with the words for God in every other language; their signification is very limited. This word *Om,* however, has around it all the various significances. As such it should be accepted by everyone.

28

The repetition of this (Om) and meditating on its meaning [is the way].

Why should there be repetition? We have not forgotten the theory of samskāras: that the sum total of impressions lives in the mind. They may become more and more latent, but they remain there, and as soon as they get the right stimulus they come out. Atomic vibration never ceases. When this universe is destroyed, all the massive vibrations disappear; the sun, moon, stars, and earth melt down; but the vibrations remain in the atoms. Each atom performs the same function as the big worlds do. So even when the vibrations of the chitta subside, its atomic vibrations go on; and when they get the impulse, they come out again.

We can now understand what is meant by repetition. It is the greatest stimulus that can be given to the spiritual samskāras. "One moment of company with the holy builds a ship to cross this ocean of life"— such is the power of association. So this repetition of Om and thinking of its meaning are the same as keeping good company in your own mind. Study and then meditate on what you have studied. Thus light will come to you; the Self will become manifest. But one must think of Om and of its meaning too.

Avoid evil company, because the scars of old wounds are in you and evil company is just the thing necessary to call them out. In the same way, we are told that good company will call out the good impressions which are in us but have become latent. There is nothing holier in the world than to keep good company, because the good impressions will then tend to come to the surface.

29

From that is gained introspection and the destruction of obstacles.

The first effect of the repetition and contemplation

of Om is that the introspective power will manifest itself more and more; all the mental and physical obstacles will begin to vanish. What are the obstacles for the yogi?

30

Disease, mental laziness, doubt, lack of enthusiasm, lethargy, clinging to sense enjoyments, false perception, non-attaining of concentration, and falling away from concentration when attained—these are the obstructing distractions.

Disease: This body is the boat which will carry us to the other shore of the ocean of life. It must be taken care of. Unhealthy persons cannot be yogis. *Mental laziness* makes us lose all lively interest in the subject, without which there will be neither the will nor the energy to practise. *Doubts* will arise in the mind about the truth of the science of Yoga, however strong one's intellectual conviction may be, until certain peculiar psychic experiences come, such as hearing or seeing at a distance. These glimpses strengthen the mind and make the student persevere. *Falling away from concentration when attained:* Some days or weeks, when you are practising, the mind will be calm and easily concentrated and you will find yourself progressing fast. All of a sudden, one day, the progress will stop and you will find yourself, as it were, stranded. But persevere. All progress proceeds by such rise and fall.

31

Grief, mental distress, tremor of the body, and

irregular breathing accompany non-retention of concentration.

Concentration will bring perfect repose to mind and body every time it is practised. When the practice has been misdirected or the mind not well controlled, these disturbances come. Repetition of Om and self-surrender to the Lord will strengthen the mind and bring fresh energy. The nervous shakings will come to almost everyone. Do not mind them at all, but keep on practising. Practice will cure them and make the seat firm.

32

To remedy this [one should] practise on one object.

Making the mind take the form of one object for some time will destroy these obstacles. This is general advice. In the following aphorisms it will be expanded and particularized. As one practice cannot suit everyone, various methods will be advanced, and everyone by actual experience will find out that which helps him most.

33

The feelings of friendship, mercy, gladness, and indifference, in regard to objects happy, unhappy, good, and evil, respectively, pacify the chitta.

We must have these four kinds of attitudes. We must have friendship for all; we must be merciful towards those that are in misery; when people are happy we ought to be happy; and to the wicked we must be indifferent. So with all objects that come before us. If the object is a good one, we must feel friendly towards it; if the object of thought is one that is miserable, we must be merciful towards the object. If it is good we must be glad; and if it is evil we must be indifferent. These attitudes of mind towards the different objects that come before it will make the mind peaceful. Most of our difficulties in our daily lives come from our being unable to hold down our minds in this way. For instance, if a man does evil to us, instantly we want to react with evil. Every reaction in the form of evil shows that we are not able to hold the chitta down; it comes out in waves towards the object, and we lose our mental power. Every reaction in the form of hatred or evil is so much loss to the mind, and every evil thought or deed of hatred, or any thought of reaction, if it is controlled, will be laid up in our favour. Not that we lose anything by thus restraining ourselves; rather we gain infinitely more than we suspect. Each time we suppress hatred or a feeling of anger, it is so much good energy stored up in our favour; that energy will be converted into the higher powers.

34

By expelling and restraining the breath [the chitta is pacified].

The word used is prāna. Prāna is not exactly breath; it is the name for the energy that pervades the universe. Whatever you see in the universe, whatever moves or works or has life, is a manifestation of prāna. The sum total of the energy displayed in the universe is called prāna. This prāna, when a cycle ends, remains in an almost motionless state, and when the next cycle begins, it gradually manifests itself. It is prāna that is manifested as motion, as the nervous motion in human beings and animals; and the same prāna is manifested as thought, and so on. The whole universe is a combination of prāna and ākāśa; so is the human body. Out of ākāśa you get the different materials that you feel and see, and out of prāna all the various forces. Now, the expelling and restraining of the prāna is what is called prānāyāma.

Patanjali, the father of the Yoga philosophy, does not give very many particular directions about prānāyāma; but later on other yogis found out various things about prānāyāma and made of it a great science. With Patanjali it is one of the many ways; but he does not lay much stress on it. He means that you simply expel the air, and draw it in, and hold it for some time—that is all; and by that the mind will become a little calmer. But you will find that out of this, later on, was evolved a particular science called prānāyāma. We shall study a little of what these later yogis have to say. Some of this I have told you before, but a little repetition will serve to fix it in your minds.

First, you must remember that prāna is not the breath; but that which causes the motion of the breath, that which is the vitality of the breath, is prāna. Again, the word *prāna* is used for all the senses; they are all called prānas; and the mind is called a prāna. We have also seen that prāna is force. And yet we cannot call it force, because force is only the manifestation of it. It is that which manifests itself as force and everything else in the shape of motion. The chitta, the mind-stuff, is an engine which draws in prāna from its surroundings and manufactures out of prāna the various vital forces—those that keep the body in preservation—and thought, will, and all other powers. By the above-mentioned process of breathing we can control all the various motions in the body, and the various nerve currents that are flowing through the body. First we begin to recognize them, and then we slowly get control over them.

Now, according to the later yogis, there are three main currents of prāna in the human body. One they call the Idā, another the Pingalā, and the third the Sushumnā. The Pingalā, according to them, is on the right side of the spinal column, and the Idā on the left, and in the middle of the spinal column is the Sushumnā, a hollow canal. The Idā and the Pingalā, according to them, are currents working in every man, and through these currents we perform all the functions of life. Though the Sushumnā is present in all, it is not active; it functions only in the yogi. You must remember that yoga changes the body; as you go on practising your body changes; it is not the same body that you had before the practice. That is very rational and can be explained. Every new thought that we entertain must make, as it were, a new channel through the brain. This explains the tremendous conservatism of human nature. Human nature likes to run through the ruts that are already there, because it is easy. If we think, just for example's sake, that the mind is like a needle, and the brain substance a soft lump before it, then each thought that we have makes a channel, as it were, in the brain. This channel would close up, but for the grey matter, which comes in and makes a lining to keep it open. If there were no grey matter there would be no memory, because memory means going over these old channels, retracing a thought, as it were. Now, perhaps you have noticed that when a man talks on subjects in which he takes up a few ideas that are familiar to everyone, and combines and recombines them, it is easy to follow him, because these channels are present in everyone's brain, and it is only necessary to refer to them. But whenever a new subject comes, new channels have to be made; so it is not readily understood. And that is why the brain (it is the brain, and not the people themselves) unconsciously refuses to be acted upon by new ideas. It resists. Prāna tries to make new channels, and the brain will not allow it. This is the secret of conservatism. The fewer channels there are in the brain and the less the needle of prāna has made these passages, the more conservative will be the brain and the more it will struggle against new thoughts. The more thoughtful the man, the more complicated will be the channels in his brain and the more easily he will take to new ideas and understand them. So with every fresh idea we make a new impression in the brain, cut new channels through the brain-stuff; and that is why we find that in the practice of yoga—consisting, as it does, of an entirely new set of thoughts and motives—there is so much physical resistance at first. That is why we find that the part of religion which deals with the external side of nature can be so widely accepted, while the other part, the philosophy or the psychology, which deals with the inner nature of man, is so frequently neglected.

We must remember the definition of this world of ours: it is only the Infinite Existence projected into the plane of consciousness. A little of the Infinite is projected into consciousness, and that we call our world. So there is an Infinite Beyond, and religion has to deal with both—with the little lump we call our world and with the Infinite Beyond. Any religion which deals with one only of these two will be defective. It must deal with both. That part of religion which deals with the part of the Infinite which has come into the plane of consciousness and got itself caught, as it were, in the plane of consciousness, in the cage of time, space, and causation, is quite familiar to us, because we are in it already, and ideas about this plane have been with us almost from time immemorial. The part of religion which deals with the Infinite Beyond comes to us entirely new, and our effort to understand produces new channels in the brain, disturbing the whole system. That is why you find that in the practice of yoga ordinary people are at first turned out of their grooves. In order to lessen these disturbances as much as possible, all these methods have been devised by Patanjali. We may practise any one which is best suited to us.

35

Those forms of concentration which bring extraordinary sense perceptions cause perseverance of the mind.

This naturally comes with dhāranā, concentration. The yogis say that if the mind is concentrated on the tip of the nose, after a few days one begins to smell wonderful perfumes. If it is concentrated on the root of the tongue, one begins to hear sounds; if on the tip of the tongue, one begins to taste wonderful flavours; if on the middle of the tongue, one feels as if one were coming in contact with some object. If one concentrates the mind on the palate one begins to see strange things. If a man whose mind is disturbed wants to take up some of these practices of yoga, yet doubts the truth of them, he will have his doubts set at rest when, after a little practice, these things come to him, and he will persevere.

36

Or [the chitta is pacified by meditation on] the Effulgent Light, which is beyond all sorrow.

This is another sort of concentration. Think of the lotus of the heart, with petals downward, and running through it, the Sushumnā. Take in the breath, and while expelling it imagine that the petals are turned upward and that inside the lotus is an effulgent light. Meditate on that.

37

Or [by meditation on] the heart that has given up all attachment to sense-objects.

Take some holy person, some great person whom you revere, some saint whom you know to be perfectly non-attached, and think of his heart. That heart has become non-attached. Meditate on that heart and it will calm the mind. If you cannot do that, there is the next way.

38

Or [by meditation on] the knowledge that comes in dreams or the happiness experienced in deep sleep.

Sometimes a man dreams that he sees angels and talks to them, and that he is in an ecstatic condition and hears music floating through the air. All this makes a deep impression on him when he awakes. Let him think of that dream as real and meditate upon it.

39

Or by meditation on anything that appeals to one as good.

This does not mean a wicked subject, but anything good that you like: the place that you like best, the scenery that you like best, the idea that you like best —anything that will concentrate the mind.

40

The yogi's mind, thus meditating, becomes unob-structed from the atomic to the infinite.

The mind, by this practice, easily contemplates the most minute as well as the biggest thing. Thus the waves of the mind become fainter.

41

The yogi whose vrittis have thus become powerless (i.e. controlled) obtains, in the receiver, [the instru-ment of] receiving, and the received (i.e. the soul, the mind, and external objects), concentratedness and sameness, like a crystal [before different coloured objects].

What results from this constant meditation? We must remember how, in a previous aphorism, we took up the various states of meditation: the first was on gross objects, the second on fine, and from them we proceeded to still finer objects. The result is that we can meditate as easily on fine as on gross objects. While meditating thus the yogi sees three things: the receiver, the received, and the receiving instrument, corresponding to the soul, external objects, and the mind. There are three objects of meditation given us: first, gross things, such as bodies or material objects; second, fine things, such as the mind, the chitta; and third, the Purusha qualified—not the Purusha Itself, but the ego. By practice the yogi gets established in all these meditations. Whenever he meditates he can keep out all other thoughts; he becomes identified with that on which he meditates. When he meditates he is like a piece of crystal. Before flowers the crystal becomes almost identified with the flowers: if the flower is red, the crystal looks red, and if the flower is blue, the crystal looks blue.

42

[The samādhi in which] sound, meaning, and the resulting knowledge are mixed is [called] "samādhi with question."

Sound here means vibration; meaning, the nerve currents which conduct it; and knowledge, the reaction. All the various meditations we have discussed so far, Patanjali calls savitarka, "with question." Later on he gives us higher and higher meditations. In these that are called "with question," we keep the duality

of subject and object, which results from the mixture
of word, meaning, and knowledge. There is first the
external vibration, the word; this, carried inward by
the nerve currents, is the meaning. After that there
comes a reactionary wave in the chitta, which is
knowledge; but the mixture of these three makes what
we call knowledge. In all the meditations up to this
we get this mixture as objects of meditation. The next
samādhi is higher.

43

The samādhi called "without question" [is attained]
when the memory is purified, or becomes devoid of
qualities, expressing only the meaning [of the object
meditated on].

It is by the practice of meditation on these three
that we come to the state where these three are not
mixed. We can get rid of them. We shall first try
to understand what these three are. Here is the chitta.
You should always remember the comparison of the
mind-stuff to a lake, and the vibration, the word, the
sound, to a wave coming over it. You have that calm
lake in you, and I pronounce a word, "cow." As soon
as it enters through your ears there is a wave produced
in your chitta along with it. So that wave represents
the idea of the cow—the form or the meaning as we
call it. The apparent cow that you know is really the
wave in the mind-stuff that comes as a reaction to the
internal and external sound vibrations. With the
sound, the wave dies away; it can never exist without
a word. You may ask what happens when we only
think of the cow and do not hear the sound. At such
times you make that sound yourself. You are saying

"cow" inaudibly in your mind, and with that comes the wave. There cannot be any wave without this impulse of sound, and when it is not from outside it is from inside; and when the sound dies, the wave dies. What remains? The result of the reaction—and that is knowledge. These three are so closely combined in our minds that we cannot separate them. When the sound comes, the senses vibrate, and the wave rises as a reaction; they follow so closely upon one another that there is no discerning one from the other. When this meditation has been practised for a long time, the memory, the receptacle of all impressions, becomes purified, and we are able to distinguish them clearly from one another. This is called nirvitarka, samādhi "without question."

44

By this process [the samādhis] "with discrimination" and "without discrimination," whose objects are finer, are [also] explained.

A process similar to the preceding is applied again; but the objects to be taken up in the former meditations are gross, whereas in this they are fine.

45

The finer objects end with the pradhāna.

The gross objects are only the elements, and everything manufactured out of them. The fine objects begin with the tanmātras, or fine particles. The organs, the mind,[2] ego, the mind-stuff (the cause of all manifestation), the state of equilibrium of sattva, rajas,

---

[2] The mind, or common sensory, the aggregate of all the senses.

and tamas—called the pradhāna (the chief), prakriti
(nature), or avyakta (the unmanifest)—are all included within the category of fine objects, the Purusha
(the Soul) alone being excepted.

46

These samādhis are "with seed."

These do not destroy the seed of past actions and
thus cannot give liberation; but what they bring to
the yogi is stated in the following aphorism.

47

When the yogi becomes established in the samādhi
"without discrimination," his chitta becomes firmly
fixed.

48

The knowledge attained through it is called
"filled with Truth."

The next aphorism will explain this.

49

The knowledge that is gained from testimony and
inference is about ordinary objects. That from the
samādhi just mentioned is of a much higher order,
being able to penetrate where inference and testimony cannot go.

The idea is that we obtain our knowledge of ordinary objects by direct perception, by inference therefrom, and through the testimony of people who are
competent. By people who are competent the yogis
always mean the rishis, the seers of the thoughts
recorded in the scriptures, the Vedas. According to

them, the only proof of the scriptures is that they were the testimony of competent persons; yet they say that the scriptures cannot take us to realization. We may read all the Vedas and yet not realize anything; but when we practise their teachings, then we shall attain to that state in which we realize what the scriptures say, which penetrates where neither reason nor perception nor inference can go, and where the testimony of others is of no avail. This is what is meant by the aphorism. Realization is the real religion; all the rest is only preparation—hearing lectures, or reading books, or reasoning, is merely preparing the ground; this is not religion. Intellectual assent and intellectual dissent are not religion.

The central idea of the yogis is that just as we come in direct contact with the objects of the senses, so also we can directly perceive religion itself, though in a far more intense sense. The truths of religion, such as God or the Soul, cannot be perceived by the external senses. I cannot see God with my eyes, nor can I touch Him with my hands. We also know that neither can we reason beyond the senses. Reason leaves us at a point quite indecisive. We may reason all our lives, as the world has been doing for thousands of years, but the only result will be that we shall find we are incompetent to prove or disprove the facts of religion. What we perceive directly we take as a basis, and upon that basis we reason. So it is obvious that reasoning has to run within the bounds of perception; it can never go beyond. The whole scope of realization, therefore, is beyond sense perception. The yogis say that man can go beyond his direct sense perception and beyond his reason also. Man has in him the faculty, the power, of transcending even his intellect —a power which is in every being, every creature. By the practice of yoga that power is aroused, and then a man transcends the ordinary limits of reason and directly perceives things which are beyond all reason.

50

The resulting impression from this samādhi obstructs all other impressions.

We have seen in the foregoing aphorism that the only way of attaining to superconsciousness is through samādhi, and we have also seen that the past samskāras, or impressions, are what hinder the mind from achieving samādhi. All of you have observed that when you are trying to concentrate your mind, your thoughts wander. When you are trying to think of God, that is the very time these samskāras appear. At other times they are not so active, but when you do not want them they are sure to be there, trying their best to crowd into your mind. Why should that be so? Why should they be much more potent at the time of concentration? It is because you are repressing them and they react with all their force. At other times they do not react. How countless these old past impressions must be, all lodged somewhere in the chitta, ready, waiting like tigers, to jump up! These have to be suppressed that the one idea which we want may arise, to the exclusion of the others. Instead they are all struggling to come up at the same time. Such is the power of the various samskāras in hindering concentration of the mind. So this samādhi which has just been given is the best to be practised, on account of its power of suppressing the samskāras. The samskāra raised by this sort of concentration will be so powerful that it will hinder the action of the others and hold them in check.

51

By the restraint of even this [impression, which obstructs all other impressions], all being restrained, comes the seedless samādhi.

You remember that our goal is to perceive the Soul Itself. We cannot perceive the Soul because It has got mixed up with nature, with the mind, with the body. The ignorant man thinks his body is the Soul. The learned man thinks his mind is the Soul. But both of them are mistaken. What makes the Soul get mixed up with all this? Different waves that rise in the chitta and cover the Soul. We see only a little reflection of the Soul through these waves; so if the wave is one of anger, we think the Soul is angry—"I am angry," we say. If it is one of love, we see ourselves reflected in that wave and say we love. If that wave is one of weakness, and the Soul is reflected in it, we think we are weak. These various ideas come from these impressions, these samskāras, covering the Soul. The real nature of the Soul is not perceived as long as there is one single wave in the lake of the chitta; this real nature will never be perceived until all the waves have subsided. So first Patanjali teaches us the meaning of these waves; secondly, the best way to repress them; and thirdly, how to make one wave so strong as to suppress all other waves, fire eating fire, as it were. When only one remains, it will be easy to suppress that also, and when that is done, the samādhi or concentration that follows is called "seedless." It leaves nothing, and the Soul is manifested just as It is, in Its own glory. Then alone do we know that the Soul is not a compound; It is the only eternally simple substance in the universe; and as such, It cannot be born, It cannot die. It is immortal, indestructible, the ever living essence of intelligence.

CONCENTRATION: ITS PRACTICE

1

Mortification, study, and the surrender of the fruits of work to God are called kriyā-yoga.

Those samādhis with which the first chapter ended are very difficult to attain; so we must take them up slowly. The first step, the preliminary step, is called kriyā-yoga. Literally, this means practising yoga through work. The organs are the horses, the mind is the reins, the intellect is the charioteer, the soul is the rider, and the body is the chariot. If the horses are very strong and do not obey the reins, and if the charioteer has no discrimination, then the rider comes to grief. But if the horses, the organs, are well controlled by the reins, the mind, and the charioteer possesses discrimination, then the rider, the soul, reaches the goal.

What is meant, in this case, by "mortification"? It means holding the reins firmly while guiding the body and the organs; not letting them do everything they like, but keeping them both under proper control.

What is meant by "study"? Not study of novels or story-books, but study of those works which teach the liberation of the soul. Then again, this study does not mean controversial studies at all. The yogi is supposed to have finished his period of controversy. He

143

has had enough of that and has become satisfied. He studies only to intensify his convictions. Vāda and siddhānta are the two kinds of scriptural knowledge: vāda, the argumentative, and siddhānta, the decisive. When a man is entirely ignorant he takes up the first of these, the argumentative, fighting and reasoning pro and con; and when he has finished that he takes up the siddhānta, the decisive, arriving at a conclusion. Simply arriving at this conclusion will not do. It must be realized. Books are infinite in number, and time is short; therefore the secret of knowledge is to take only what is essential. Take what is essential and try to live up to it. There is an old Indian legend that if you place a cup of milk and water before a rāja-hamsa, a swan, he will take all the milk and leave the water. In that way we should take what is of value in knowledge and leave the dross. Intellectual gymnastics are necessary at first; we must not go blindly into anything. But the yogi has passed the argumentative stage and has come to a conclusion, which is immovable, like the rocks. The only thing he now seeks to do is to intensify that conclusion. Do not argue, he says; if anyone forces arguments upon you, be silent. Do not answer any argument, but go away calmly, because arguments only disturb the mind. The only use of argument is to train the intellect. When that is accomplished, what is the use of disturbing it further? The intellect is but a weak instrument and can only give us knowledge limited by the senses. The yogi wants to go beyond the senses; therefore the intellect is of no ultimate use to him. He is certain of this and therefore is silent and does not argue. Every argument throws his mind out of balance, creates a disturbance in the chitta; and a disturbance is a drawback. Argumentation and reasoning are only preliminary stages; there are things beyond them. The whole of life is not for schoolboy fights and debating societies.

The "surrender of the fruits of work to God" means to take to ourselves neither credit nor blame, but to give both up to the Lord and be at peace.

2

[Kriyā-yoga leads to] samādhi and attenuates the pain-bearing obstructions.

Most of us are spoilt children, who allow the mind to do whatever it wants. Therefore it is necessary that kriyā-yoga should be constantly practised, in order to gain control of the mind and bring it into subjection. The obstructions to yoga arise from lack of control and cause us pain. They can be removed only by controlling the mind and holding it in check through kriyā-yoga.

3

The pain-bearing obstructions are ignorance, egoity, attachment, aversion, and clinging to life.

These are the five kinds of pain, the fivefold tie that binds us down. Of them, ignorance is the cause, and the other four are the effects. It is the only cause of all our misery. What else can make us miserable? The nature of the Soul is eternal bliss. What can make It sorrowful except ignorance, hallucination, delusion? All pain in the Soul is simply delusion.

4

Ignorance is the productive field of all those that
follow, whether they are dormant, attenuated, overpowered, or expanded.

Ignorance is the cause of egoity, attachment, aversion, and clinging to life. These impressions exist in
different states. They are sometimes dormant. You
often hear the expression "innocent as a baby"; yet
in the baby may be the nature of a demon, which
will come out by degrees. In the yogi, these impressions, the samskāras left by past actions, are "attenuated," that is, their power is much weakened;
and he can control them and not allow them to become manifest. "Overpowered" means that sometimes
one set of impressions is held down for a while by
those that are stronger; but they come out when that
repressing cause is removed. The last state is the "expanded," when the samskāras, having helpful surroundings, attain to great activity, either as good or
evil.

5

Ignorance is to take what is non-eternal, impure,
painful, and not-Self, for what is eternal, pure,
happy and the Ātman, or Self, [respectively].

All the different sorts of impressions have one
source: ignorance. We have first to learn what ignorance is. Every one of us thinks: "I am the body, and
not the Self, the pure, the effulgent, the ever blissful"
—and that is ignorance. We think of the Self and see
It as the body. This is the great delusion.

6

Egoity is the identification of the Seer with the instrument of seeing.

The Seer is really the Self, the Pure One, the Ever Holy, the Infinite, the Immortal. This is the Self of man. And what are the instruments? The chitta, or mind-stuff, the buddhi, or determinative faculty, the manas, or mind, and the indriyas, or sense-organs. These are Its instruments for seeing the external world; and the identification of the Self with the instruments is what is called egoity, which results from ignorance. We say: "I am the mind," "I am unhappy," "I am angry," or "I am happy." How can we be angry and how can we hate? We should identify ourselves with 'the Self; That cannot change. If It is unchangeable, how can It be one moment happy and one moment unhappy? It is formless, infinite, omnipresent. What can change It? It is beyond all law. What can affect It? Nothing in the universe can produce an effect on It; yet, through ignorance, we identify ourselves with the mind-stuff and think we feel pleasure or pain.

7

Attachment is that which dwells on pleasure.

We find pleasure in certain things, and the mind, like a current, flows towards them; and this following the centre of pleasure, as it were, is what is called attachment. We are never attached to that in which we do not find pleasure. We find pleasure in very queer things, sometimes, but the principle remains that whatever object we find pleasure in, to that we are attached.

8

Aversion is that which dwells on pain.

That which gives us pain we immediately seek to get away from.

9

Abiding in its own nature [due to the past experience of death], and established even in the learned, is the clinging to life.

This clinging to life you see manifested in every living being. Upon it attempts have been made to build the theory of a future life, because men are so fond of life that they desire a future life also. Of course, it goes without saying that this argument is without much value; but the most curious part of it is that in Western countries the idea that this clinging to life indicates a possibility of future life applies only to men but does not include animals.

In India this clinging to life has been one of the arguments to prove past experience and existence. For instance, if it is true that all our knowledge has come from experience, then it is sure that that which we never experienced we cannot imagine or understand. As soon as chickens are hatched they begin to pick up food. Many times it has been seen that, when ducks have been hatched by a hen, they run to the water as soon as they come out of the eggs, and the mother hen thinks they will drown. If experience is the only source of knowledge, where do chickens learn to pick up food, or ducklings learn that water is their natural element? If you say it is instinct, it means nothing; it is simply giving a word, but is no explanation. What is this instinct? We have many instincts in ourselves. For instance, those of you who play the piano can remember, when you first were learning, how carefully you had to put your fingers on the black and the white keys, one after the other, but now, after long years of practice, you can talk with your friends while your fingers play mechanically. Your playing has become instinctive. So with every work: by practice it becomes instinctive and automatic, and so far as we know, all the cases which we now regard as automatic are degenerated reason. In the language of the yogi, instinct is involved reason. Discrimination becomes involved and gets to be automatic samskāras. Therefore it is perfectly logical to think that all that we call instinct in this world is simply involved reason. As reason cannot come without experience, all instinct is, therefore, the result of past experience. Chickens fear the hawk, and ducklings love the water; these are both the results of past experience.

Then the question is whether that experience belongs to a particular soul or simply to the body, whether this experience which comes to the duck is the duck's forefathers' experience or the duck's own experience. Modern scientific men hold that it belongs to the body; but the yogis hold that it is the experience of the mind, transmitted through the body. This is called the theory of reincarnation. We have seen that all our knowledge, whether we call it perception or reason or instinct, must come through that one channel called experience, and that all that we now call instinct is the result of past experience, degenerated into instinct, and that instinct regenerates into reason again. And this is so throughout the universe. Upon this, in India, has been built one of the chief arguments for reincarnation.

The recurring experience of various fears produces, in course of time, this clinging to life. That is why the child is instinctively afraid; the past experience of pain is there in it. Even in the most learned men, who know that this body will die and who say: "Never mind. We have had hundreds of bodies; the Soul cannot die"—even in them, with all their intellectual conviction, we still find this clinging to life. Why is there this clinging to life? We have seen that it has become instinctive. In the psychological language of the yogis it has become a samskāra. The samskāras, fine and hidden, are sleeping in the chitta. All these past experiences of death, all that we call instinct, are experiences become subconscious. They live in the chitta; and they are not inactive, but work underneath.

The chitta-vrittis, the mind-waves, which are gross, we can appreciate and feel; they can be more easily controlled. But what about the finer instincts? How can they be controlled? When I am angry my whole mind becomes a huge wave of anger. I feel it, see it, handle it, can easily manipulate it, can fight with it; but I shall not succeed completely in the fight until I can get down to its causes. A man says something very harsh to me, and I begin to feel that I am getting heated; and he goes on till I am totally angry, till I forget myself and identify myself with anger. When he first began to abuse me, I thought, "I am going to be angry"; the anger was one thing and I was another. But when I became angry, I was the anger. These feelings have to be controlled in the germ, the root, in their fine forms, even before we have become conscious that they are acting on us. With the majority of mankind the fine states of these passions are not even known—the states below consciousness from which they slowly emerge. When a bubble is rising from the bottom of the lake we do not see it, nor even when it has nearly come to the surface; it is only when it bursts and makes a ripple that we know it is there. We shall only be successful in grappling with the waves when we can get hold of them in their fine forms; until we can get hold of them and subdue them before they become gross, there is no hope of conquering any passion perfectly. To control our passions we have to control them at their very root; then alone shall we be able to burn out their seeds. As fried seeds sown in the ground will never come up, so these passions will never arise.

10

The fine samskāras are to be conquered by resolving them into their causal state.

The samskāras are the subtle impressions which remain even when the mental waves are destroyed by meditation. How can these samskāras be controlled? By resolving the effect into the cause. When the chitta, which is an effect, is resolved, through samādhi, into its cause, asmitā or "I-consciousness," then only do the fine impressions die along with it.

11

By meditation their [gross] modifications are to be rejected.

Meditation is one of the effective means of controlling the rise of these waves. By meditation you can subdue these mental waves; and if you go on practising meditation for days and months and years—until it has become a habit, until it comes in spite of yourself —anger and hatred will be completely controlled and checked.

12

The "receptacle of works" has its roots in the aforesaid pain-bearing obstructions, and the experience of the latter is in this visible (present) life or in the unseen (next) life.

By the "receptacle of works" is meant the sum total of samskāras. Any work we do throws the mind into a wave; and after the work is finished we think the wave is gone. But it is not so; the wave has only become fine; it is still there. When we try to remember the work, it comes up again and becomes a wave. So it is there; if not, there would not have been memory. Thus every action, every thought, good or bad, goes into the deepest level of the mind, becomes fine, and remains stored up there. Both happy and unhappy thoughts are called "pain-bearing obstructions," because, according to the yogis, in the long run both bring pain. All happiness which comes from the senses will eventually bring pain. All enjoyment will make us thirst for more, and that brings pain as its result.

There is no limit to man's desire; he goes on desiring, and when he comes to a point where desire cannot be fulfilled, the result is pain. Therefore the yogis regard the sum total of the impressions, good or evil, as pain-bearing obstructions; they obstruct the way to the freedom of the Soul.

The samskāras, the fine roots of all our works, should be regarded as causes which will bring effects either in this life or in the lives to come. In exceptional cases, when these samskāras are very strong, they bear fruit quickly; exceptional acts of wickedness or of goodness bring their fruits even in this life. The yogis hold that men who are able while living to acquire a tremendous power of good samskāras do not have to die, but even in this life can change their bodies into god bodies. There are several such cases mentioned by the yogis in their books. These men change the very material of their bodies; they rearrange the molecules in such a fashion that they have no more sickness, and what we call death does not come to them. Why should this not be? Physiologically, the eating of food means assimilation of energy from the sun. The energy first enters the plant, the plant is eaten by an animal, and the animal by a man. This means, in the language of science, that we take an amount of energy from the sun and make it part of ourselves. If that be so, why should there be only one way of assimilating energy? The plant's way is not the same as ours; the earth's process of assimilating energy differs from our own. But all assimilate energy in some way or other. The yogis contend that they are able to assimilate energy by the power of the mind alone, that they can

draw in as much of it as they desire without recourse
to the ordinary methods. As a spider makes its web
out of its own substance, and becomes bound by it,
and cannot go anywhere except along the lines of that
web, so we have projected out of the material of our
bodies this network called the nerves, and now we
cannot work except through the channels of those
nerves. The yogis say that we need not be bound by
them.

To give another example, we can send electricity to
any part of the world, but we have to send it by means
of wires. Nature can send a vast mass of electricity
without any wires at all. Why cannot we do the same?
We can send mental electricity everywhere. What we
call mind is very much the same as electricity. It is
clear that the nerve fluid has some amount of electricity, because it is polarized and has all the char-
acteristics of electricity. We can now send our electricity only through these nerve channels. Why can we
not send mental electricity without this aid? The yogis
say that it is perfectly possible and practicable, and
that when you can do that you will work all over the
universe. You will be able to work with any body anywhere, without the help of the nervous system. When
the soul is acting through these nerve channels we
say that a man is living, and when it ceases to work
through them a man is said to be dead. But when a
man can act either with or without these channels,
birth and death will have no meaning for him. All the
bodies in the universe are made up of tanmātras; their
difference lies in the arrangement of the latter. If you
are the arranger you can arrange a body in one way or

another. Who makes up this body but you? Who eats the food? If another ate the food for you, you would not live long. Who makes the blood out of the food? You, certainly. Who purifies the blood and sends it through the veins? You. We are the masters of the body and we live in it. Only we have lost the knowledge of how to rejuvenate it; we have become automatic, degenerate; we have forgotten the process of arranging its molecules. So what we do automatically has to be done knowingly. We are the masters and we have to regulate that arrangement, and as soon as we can do that we shall be able to rejuvenate ourselves just as we like, and then we shall have neither birth nor disease nor death.

13

The roots being there, the fruition comes in [the form of] species, longevity, and experience of pleasure and pain.

The roots, the causes, the samskāras being there, in the mind, they manifest themselves and form the effects. The cause dying down becomes the effect; the effect getting subtler becomes the cause of the next effect. A tree bears a seed, which becomes the cause of another tree, and so on. All our present works are the effects of past samskāras; again, these works, becoming samskāras, will be the causes of future actions, and thus we go on. So this aphorism says that, the causes being there, the fruit must come in the form of species of beings: one will be a man, another an angel, another an animal, another a demon. Then there are different effects of karma on longevity: one man lives fifty years, another a hundred, another dies in two years and never attains maturity. All these differences in longevity are regulated by past karma. One man is born, as it were, for pleasure; if he buries himself in a forest, pleasure will follow him there. Another man, wherever he goes, is followed by pain; everything becomes painful for him. It is all the result of their own past. According to the philosophy of the yogis, all virtuous actions bring pleasure and all vicious actions bring pain. Any man who does wicked deeds is sure to reap their fruit in the form of pain.

14

They (i.e. actions) bear fruit as pleasure or pain, caused by virtue or vice.

15

To the discriminating, all is, as it were, painful because everything brings pain, either as consequence or as anticipation of loss of happiness or as fresh craving arising from impressions of happiness, and also because the gunas counteract one another.

The yogis say that the man who has the power of discrimination, the man of good sense, sees through all that is called pleasure or pain and knows that they come to all, and that one follows and melts into the other. He sees that men follow an ignis fatuus all their lives and never succeed in fulfilling their desires. The great king Yudhishthira once said that the most wonderful thing in life is that every moment we see people dying around us and yet we think we shall never die. We think that, though surrounded by fools on every side, we are the only exceptions, the only learned men. Though everywhere we experience fickleness, we think our love is the only lasting love. How can that be? Even love is selfish; and the yogi says that in the end we shall find that even the love of husbands and wives and children and friends slowly decays. Decadence seizes everything in this life. It is only when everything, even love, fails that, in a flash, man finds out how vain, how dreamlike, is this world. Then he catches a glimpse of vairāgya, renunciation, catches a glimpse of the Beyond. It is only by giving up this world that the other is seen—never through holding on to this one. Never yet was there a great soul who had not to reject sense pleasures and enjoyments to acquire his greatness. The cause of misery is the clash between the different forces (gunas) of nature, one dragging one way and another dragging another, rendering permanent happiness impossible.

16

The misery which has not yet come is to be avoided.

Some karma we have worked out already, some we are working out in our present life, and some is waiting to bear fruit in a future life. The first kind is past and gone. The second we shall have to work out. It is only that which is waiting to bear fruit in the future that we can conquer and control; and towards this end all our forces should be directed. This is what Patanjali means when he says (II. 10.) that the samskāras are to be controlled by resolving them into their causal state.

17

The cause of that [misery] which is to be avoided is the junction of the Seer and the seen.

Who is the Seer? The Self of man, the Purusha. What is the seen? The whole of nature, from the mind down to gross matter. All pleasure and pain arise from the joining of the Purusha and the mind. The Purusha, you must remember, according to this philosophy is pure; when joined to nature, and reflected therein, It appears to feel pleasure or pain.

18

The seen, which is composed of elements and organs, and characterized by illumination, action, and inertia, is for the purpose of experience and release [of the Seer].

Nature, or the seen, is composed of gross and fine elements and the organs—that is to say, the sense-organs, the mind, and so forth—and is characterized by illumination (sattva), action (rajas), and inertia (tamas). What is the whole purpose of the seen, or nature? It is to give the Purusha experience. The Purusha has, as it were, forgotten Its mighty, godlike nature. There is a story that the king of the gods, Indra, once became a pig wallowing in mire; he had a she-pig and a lot of baby pigs and was very happy. Then some gods saw his plight and came to him and said, "You are the king of the gods; you have all the gods under your command; why are you here?" But Indra said: "Never mind. I am all right here; I do not care for heaven while I have this sow and these little pigs." The poor gods were at their wits' end. After a time they decided to slay all the pigs one after another. When all were dead, Indra began to weep and mourn. Then the gods ripped his pig body open, and he came out of it and began to laugh when he realized what a hideous dream he had had—he, the king of the gods, to have become a pig and to have thought that that pig life was the only life! Not only so, but to have wanted the whole universe to join him in the pig life!

Likewise, the Purusha, when identified with nature, forgets that It is pure and infinite. The Purusha does not love; It is love itself. It does not exist; It is existence itself. The Soul does not know; It is knowledge itself. It is a mistake to say that the Soul loves, exists, or knows. Love, existence, and knowledge are not the qualities of the Purusha, but Its essence. When they are reflected upon something, you may call them the qualities of that thing. They are not the qualities but the essence of the Purusha, the great Ātman, the Infinite Being, without birth or death, established in Its own glory. It appears to have become so degenerate that if you come and tell It, "You are not a pig," It begins to squeal and bite.

Thus is it with us all in this māyā, this dream-world, where it is all misery, weeping, and crying, where a few golden balls are rolled and the world scrambles after them. You were never bound by laws; nature never put a bond on you. That is what the yogi tells you. Have patience to learn it. And the yogi shows how, by junction with nature, by identifying Itself with the mind and the world, the Purusha thinks Itself miserable. Then he goes on to show you that the way out is through experience. You have to get all this experience; but finish it quickly. We have placed ourselves in this net and we shall have to get out. We have got ourselves caught in the trap, and we shall have to work out our freedom. So get this experience of husbands and wives and friends and little loves; you will pass through them safely if you never forget what you really are. Never forget that this is only a momentary state and that you have to pass through it. Experience is the one great teacher—experience of pleasure and pain—but know that it is only momentary. It leads step by step to that state where all things become small, and the Purusha so great that the whole universe seems as a drop in the ocean and falls off by its own nothingness. We have to go through different experiences, but let us never forget the ideal.

19

The states of the gunas are the defined (the gross elements), the undefined (the subtle elements), the merely indicated (the cosmic intelligence), and the signless (prakriti).

The system of Yoga is built entirely on the philosophy of Sāmkhya, as I told you before; and here again I shall remind you of the cosmology of the Sāmkhya philosophy. According to Sāmkhya, nature is both the material and the efficient cause of the universe. In nature there are three gunas, or elements: sattva, rajas, and tamas. Tamas is all that is dark, all that is ignorant and heavy; rajas is activity; and sattva is calmness, light. Nature, before creation, is called avyakta, undefined or indiscrete—that is, the state in which there is no distinction of form or name, in which these three gunas are held in perfect balance. Then the balance is disturbed, the three gunas begin to mingle in various fashions, and the result is the universe.

In every man, also, these three gunas exist. When sattva prevails, knowledge comes; when rajas, activity; and when tamas, there come darkness, lassitude, idleness, and ignorance. According to the Sāmkhya theory, the highest manifestation of nature, consisting of these three gunas, is called mahat, or intelligence, universal intelligence, of which the human intellect is a part. In the Sāmkhya psychology there is a sharp distinction between the function of the manas, or mind, and the function of the buddhi, or intellect. The mind's function is simply to collect outer impressions and present them to the buddhi, the individual mahat, which decides about them. Out of mahat comes egoity, from which, again, come the subtle elements. The subtle elements combine and become the gross materials, the external universe. The claim of the Sāmkhya philosophy is that, from the intellect down to a block of stone, all things are the products of one substance, differing only as finer or grosser states of existence. The finer are the causes, and the grosser are the effects. According to the Sāmkhya philosophy, beyond the whole of nature is the Purusha, which is not material at all. The Purusha is not similar to anything else, either the buddhi or the mind or the tanmātras or the gross materials. It is not akin to any one of these; It

is entirely separate, entirely different in Its nature;
and further, it is argued that the Purusha must be
immortal, because It is not the result of combination.
That which is not the result of combination cannot
die. According to Sāmkhya, Purushas are infinite in
number.

Now we shall understand the aphorism when it says
that the states of the gunas are the defined, the undefined, the merely indicated, and the signless. By
the "defined" are meant the gross elements, which we
can sense. By the "undefined" are meant the very fine
materials, the tanmātras, which cannot be sensed by
ordinary men. If you practise yoga, however, says
Patanjali, after a while your perceptions will become
so fine that you will actually see the tanmātras. For
instance, you have heard that every man sheds a
certain light about him; every living being emits a
certain light, and this, the yogi says, can be seen by
him. We do not all see it, but we all throw out these
tanmātras, just as a flower continuously sends out the
fine particles which enable us to smell it. Every day of
our lives we throw out a mass of good or evil, and
everywhere we go the atmosphere is full of these materials. That is how there came to the human mind,
unconsciously, the idea of building temples and
churches. Why should men build churches in which
to worship God? Why not worship Him anywhere?
Even if they did not know the reason, men found that
a place where people worshipped God became full of
good tanmātras. Every day people go there, and the
more they go the holier they get and the holier that
place becomes. If any man who has not much sattva

in him goes there, the place will influence him and arouse his sattva quality. Here, therefore, is the significance of all temples and holy places; but you must remember that their holiness depends on holy people's congregating there. The difficulty with man is that he forgets the original meaning and puts the cart before the horse. It was men who made these places holy, and then the effect became the cause and made men holy. If the wicked alone were to go there it would become as bad as any other place. It is not the building, but the people, that make a church; and that is what we always forget. That is why sages and holy persons, who have much of this sattva quality, can send it out and exert a tremendous influence day and night on their surroundings. A man may be so pure that his purity will become tangible. Whosoever comes in contact with him will become pure.

Next, the "merely indicated" means the cosmic buddhi, the cosmic intellect. It is the first manifestation of nature; from it all other manifestations proceed.

Last, the "signless," or nature. There seems to be a great difference between modern science and the religions at this point. Every religion says that the universe comes out of intelligence. The theory of God, taking the word in its psychological significance, apart from all ideas of personality, is that intelligence comes first in the order of creation and that out of intelligence comes what we call gross matter. Modern scientists say that intelligence is the last to come. They say that unintelligent things slowly evolve into animals, and animals into men. They claim that instead of everything's coming out of intelligence, intelligence itself is the last to come. Both the religious and the scientific statements, though seeming to be directly opposed to each other, are true. Take an infinite series: A—B—A—B—A—B and so on. The question is: Which is first, A or B? If you take the series as A—B, you will say that A is first; but if you take it as B—A, you will say that B is first. It depends upon the way you look at it. Intelligence undergoes modification and becomes gross matter; this again becomes intelligence; and thus the process goes on. The followers of Sāmkhya, and other religious people, put intelligence first, and the series becomes intelligence, and then matter. The scientific man puts his finger on matter and says that first comes matter, and then intelligence. They both indicate the same chain. Hindu philosophy, however, goes beyond both intelligence and matter, and finds a Purusha, or Self, which is beyond intelligence, and of which intelligence is but the borrowed light.

20

The Seer is intelligence only, and though pure, sees through the colouring of the intellect.

This is again Sāmkhya philosophy. We have seen from the same philosophy that, from the lowest form up to intelligence, all is nature; beyond nature are Purushas, which have no qualities. Then how does a Purusha appear to be happy or unhappy? By reflection. If a red flower is put near a piece of pure crystal, the crystal appears to be red. Similarly, the appearance of happiness or unhappiness in the Soul is but a reflection; the Soul Itself has no colouring. The Soul is separate from nature; nature is one thing, the Soul another, eternally separate. Sāmkhya says that intelligence is a compound, that it grows and wanes, that it changes just as the body changes, and that its nature is nearly the same as that of the body. As a finger-nail is to the body, so is the body to intelligence. The nail is a part of the body, but it can be pared off hundreds of times and the body will still last. Similarly, intelligence lasts aeons, while this body can be pared off, thrown off. Yet intelligence cannot be immortal, because it changes, growing and waning. Anything that changes cannot be immortal. Certainly intelligence is manufactured; and that very fact shows us that there must be something beyond it. It cannot be free; everything connected with matter is in nature, and therefore bound for ever. Who is free? The free must certainly be beyond cause and effect.

If you say that the idea of freedom is a delusion, I shall say that the idea of bondage is also a delusion. Two facts come into our consciousness and stand or fall with each other. These are our notions of bondage and freedom. If we want to go through a wall, and our heads bump against it, we see that we are limited by that wall. At the same time, we find that we have a will-power and think we can direct our will everywhere. At every step these contradictory ideas come to us. We have to believe that we are free, yet at every moment we find we are not free. If one idea is a delusion, the other is also a delusion, and if one is true, the other also is true, because both stand upon the same basis: experience.

The yogi says that both are true—that we are bound so far as intelligence is concerned, but that we are

free so far as the Soul is concerned. The real nature
of the Soul, or Purusha, is beyond the law of causation. Its freedom is percolating through layers of
matter in various forms, through intelligence, mind,
and so forth. It is Its light that is shining through all.
Intelligence has no light of its own. Each organ has a
particular centre in the brain. There is not just one
centre for all the organs; each organ is separate. Why
do all perceptions harmonize? Where do they get their
unity? If it were in the brain, it would be necessary
for all the organs—the eyes, the nose, the ears, and
so forth—to have one centre only; whereas we know
for certain that there are different centres for each.
But a man can see and hear at the same time; so there
must be a unity at the back of intelligence. Intelligence
is connected with the brain, but behind even intelligence stands the Purusha, the Unit, where all the
different sensations and perceptions join and become
one. The Soul Itself is the centre where all the different perceptions converge and become unified. That
Soul is free, and it is Its freedom that tells you every
moment that you are free, and not bound. But you
mistakenly identify that freedom with intelligence
and mind. You try to attribute that freedom to the
intellect, and immediately find that the intellect is not
free; you attribute that freedom to the body, and
immediately nature tells you that you are again mistaken. That is why there is this mingled sense of
freedom and bondage at the same time. The yogi
analyses both what is free and what is bound, and his
ignorance vanishes. He finds that the Purusha is free,
is the essence of that knowledge which, coming

through the buddhi, becomes intelligence and, as such, is bound.

21

The [transformation that takes place in the] nature of the seen (i.e. prakriti) is for Him (i.e. the Purusha).

Prakriti has no power of its own. As long as the Purusha is near it, it appears to have power; but the power is borrowed, just as the moon's light is borrowed. According to the yogis, the whole manifested universe has come from prakriti itself; but prakriti has no purpose except to free the Purusha.

22

Though destroyed for him whose goal has been gained, yet prakriti is not destroyed for others, being common to them.

The whole activity of nature is to make the Soul know that It is entirely separate from nature. When the Soul knows this, nature has no more attractions for It. But the whole of nature vanishes only for that man who has become free. There will always remain an infinite number of others for whom nature will go on working.

23

Junction [of prakriti and the Purusha] is the cause of the realization of the nature of the powers of both the seen and its Lord.

According to this aphorism, the powers of both Soul and nature (i.e. the experiencer and the experienced) become manifest when they (i.e. the Soul and nature) are in conjunction. It is then that the manifestation of the phenomenal universe occurs. Ignorance is the cause of this conjunction. We see every day that the cause of our pain or pleasure is always our joining ourselves with the body. If I were perfectly certain that I am not this body, I should take no notice of heat and cold, or anything of the kind. This body is a combination. It is only a fiction to say that I have one body, you another, and the sun another. The whole universe is one ocean of matter, and you are the name of a little particle, and I of another, and the sun of a third. We know that this matter is continuously changing. What forms the sun one day, the next day may form the material of our bodies.

24

Ignorance is its cause.

Through ignorance we have joined ourselves with particular bodies and thus opened ourselves to misery. This idea of the body is simply a superstition. It is superstition that makes us happy or unhappy; it is superstition caused by ignorance that makes us feel heat and cold, pain and pleasure. It is our duty to rise above this superstition; and the yogi shows us how we can do this. It has been demonstrated that under certain mental conditions a man may be burnt and yet feel no pain. But this sudden exaltation of the mind comes like a whirlwind one minute and goes away the next. If, however, we gain it through yoga, we shall permanently achieve the separation of the Self from the body.

25

**There being absence of that (i.e. ignorance), there
is absence of junction. This is the destruction of
ignorance, and this is the independence of the Seer.**

According to the Yoga philosophy, it is through
ignorance that the soul has been joined with nature.
The aim is to get rid of nature's control over us. That
is the goal of all religions. Each soul is potentially
divine. The goal is to manifest this divinity within by
controlling nature: external and internal. Do this either
by work, or worship, or psychic control, or philosophy
—by one, or more, or all of these—and be free. This
is the whole of religion. Doctrines, or dogmas, or
rituals, or books, or temples, or forms, are but secondary details.

The yogi tries to reach this goal through psychic
control. Until we can free ourselves from nature we
are slaves; as it dictates so we must do. The yogi
claims that he who controls mind controls matter also.
Internal nature is much subtler than external, and
much more difficult to grapple with, much more
difficult to control. Therefore he who has conquered
internal nature controls the whole universe; it becomes his servant. Rāja-yoga propounds the methods of
gaining this control. Forces subtler than any we know
in physical nature will have to be subdued. This body
is just the external crust of the mind. They are not
two different things; they are just like the oyster and
its shell. They are but two aspects of one thing. The
internal substance of the oyster takes up matter from
outside and manufactures the shell. In the same way

the internal, fine forces which constitute the mind take up gross matter from outside and from that manufacture this external shell, the body. If, then, we have control of the internal, it is very easy to have control of the external. Then again, these forces are not different. It is not that some forces are physical, and some mental; the physical forces are but the gross manifestations of the fine forces, just as the physical world is but the gross manifestation of the fine world.

26

The means of destruction of ignorance is unbroken practice of discrimination.

This is the real goal of practice: discrimination between the real and the unreal, knowing that the Purusha is not nature, that It is neither matter nor mind, and that because It is not nature, It cannot possibly change. It is only nature which changes, combining and recombining, dissolving continually. When through constant practice we begin to discriminate, ignorance will vanish and the Purusha will begin to shine in Its real nature, omniscient, omnipotent, omnipresent.

27

His knowledge is attained in seven supreme steps.

When this knowledge comes, it comes, as it were, in seven steps, one after another; as we attain one of these we know that we are getting knowledge. The first step will make us feel that we have known what is to be known. The mind will cease to be dissatisfied. As long as we are aware of a thirst after knowledge we seek it here and there, wherever we think we can get some truth, and failing to find it we become dissatisfied and seek in a fresh direction. All search is vain until we begin to perceive that knowledge is within ourselves, that no one can help us, that we must help ourselves. When we begin to develop the power of discrimination, the first sign that we are getting near truth will be that this dissatisfied state will vanish. We shall feel quite sure that we have found the truth and that it cannot be anything else but the truth. Then we may know that the sun is rising, that the morning is breaking for us; and taking courage, we must persevere until the goal is reached.

The second step will be the absence of all pain. It will be impossible for anything in the universe, external or internal, to give us pain. The third will be the attainment of full knowledge. Omniscience will be ours. The fourth will be the attainment, through discrimination, of the end of all duties. Next will come what is called freedom of the chitta. We shall realize that all difficulties and struggles, all vacillations of the mind, have fallen away, just like a stone rolling from the mountain top into the valley and never coming up again. The next will be that the chitta will realize that it can melt away into its causes whenever we so desire.

Lastly, we shall find that we are established in our true Self, that the Self in us has existed alone throughout the universe, and that neither body nor mind has ever been related, much less joined, to It. They were working their own way, and we, through ignorance, joined the Self to them. But we have existed alone, omnipotent, omnipresent, ever blessed; our own Self was so pure and perfect that we required none else. We required none else to make us happy, for we are happiness itself. We shall find that this knowledge does not depend on anything else. Throughout the universe there can be nothing that will not become effulgent before this knowledge. This will be the last step, and the yogi will become peaceful and calm, never to feel any more pain, never again to be deluded, never to be touched by misery. He will know that he is ever blessed, ever perfect, almighty.

28

Through the practice of the different parts of yoga the impurities are destroyed and knowledge is kindled, leading up to discrimination.

Now come the practical disciplines. What we have just been speaking about is very difficult; it is far above our heads. But it is the ideal. The first thing necessary is to obtain control of the body and mind. Then the realization of the ideal will become easy. The ideal being known, what now remains is to practise the method of reaching it.

29

Yama, niyama, āsana, prānāyāma, pratyāhāra, dhāranā, dhyāna, and samādhi are the eight limbs of yoga.

30

Non-killing, truthfulness, non-stealing, continence, and non-receiving [of gifts] are called yama.

A man who wants to be a perfect yogi must give up ideas of sex. The Soul has no sex: why should It degrade Itself with ideas of sex? Later on we shall understand better why these ideas must be given up. The mind of the man who receives gifts is acted on by the mind of the giver; so the receiver is likely to become degenerate. The receiving of gifts tends to destroy the independence of the mind and make us slavish. Therefore receive no gifts.

31

These, unbroken by time, place, purpose, or caste-rules, are universal, great vows.

These disciplines—non-killing, truthfulness, non-stealing, chastity, and non-receiving—are to be practised by every yogi—man, woman, or child; by every-one, irrespective of nation, country, or position.

32

Internal and external purification, contentment, mortification, study, and worship of God are the niyamas.

External purification means keeping the body pure; a dirty man will never be a yogi. There must be in-ternal purification also. That is obtained through the practice of the virtues named in I. 33. Of course, the internal purity is of greater value than the external; but both are necessary, and the external purity, with-out the internal, is of no value.

33

When thoughts obstructive to yoga arise, contrary thoughts should be employed.

That is the way to practise the virtues that have been mentioned. For instance, when a big wave of anger has come into the mind, how are we to control it? By raising an opposing wave. Think of love. Sometimes a mother is very angry with her husband, and while she is in that state, the baby comes in and she kisses the baby; the old wave dies out and a new wave arises—love for the child. That suppresses the other one. Love is the opposite of anger. Similarly, when the idea of stealing comes, non-stealing should be thought of; when the idea of receiving gifts comes, replace it by a contrary thought.

34

The obstructions to yoga are killing, falsehood, and so forth—whether committed, caused, or approved—either through avarice, anger, or ignorance —whether slight, middling, or great; they result in infinite ignorance and misery: this is [the method of] thinking the contrary.

To tell a lie, or cause another to tell one, or to approve of another's doing so—it is all equally sinful. A very mild lie is still a lie. Every vicious thought will rebound, every thought of hatred which you may have cherished, even in a cave, is stored up and will one day come back to you with tremendous power in the form of some misery here. If you project hatred and jealousy, they will rebound on you with compound interest. No power can avert them; when once you have put them in motion you will have to bear their fruit. Remembering this will prevent you from doing wicked things.

35

When the yogi is established in non-killing, all enmities [in others] cease in his presence.

If a man realizes the ideal of not injuring others, before him even animals which are by nature ferocious will become peaceful. The tiger and the lamb will play together before that yogi. When you have come to this state, then alone will you understand that you have become firmly established in non-injury.

36

By being established in truthfulness, the yogi gets the power of attaining for himself and others the fruits of work without the work.

When this power of truth is established within you, then you will never tell an untruth even in a dream. You will be true in thought, word, and deed. Whatever you say will be truth. You may say to a man, "Be blessed," and that man will be blessed. If a man is diseased and you say to him, "Be thou cured," he will be cured immediately.

37

By being established in non-stealing, the yogi obtains all wealth.

The more you fly from nature, the more it follows you; and if you do not care for it at all, it becomes your slave.

38

By being established in continence, the yogi gains energy.

The chaste person has tremendous energy and gigantic will-power. Without chastity there can be no spiritual strength. Continence gives wonderful control over mankind. The spiritual leaders of men have been continent, and this is what gave them power. Therefore the yogi must be continent.

39

When the yogi is established in non-receiving he gets the memory of past life.

When a man does not receive presents, he is not beholden to others but remains independent and free. His mind becomes pure. With every gift, he is likely to receive the evils of the giver. If he does not receive gifts, his mind is purified, and the first power he gets is memory of past life. Then alone does the yogi become perfectly fixed in his ideal. He sees that he has been coming and going many times; so he becomes determined that this time he will be free, that he will no more come and go and be the slave of nature.

40

When he is established in internal and external cleanliness, there arises in him disgust for his own body and desire for non-intercourse with others.

When there is real purification of the body, external and internal, there arises neglect of the body; the idea of keeping it nice vanishes. A face which others call most beautiful will appear to the yogi as merely an animal face if the Spirit is not behind it. What the world calls a very common face he will regard as heavenly if the Spirit shines behind it. The thirst after the body is the great bane of human life. So the first sign of the attainment of purity is that you do not care to think you are a body. It is only when purity comes that we get rid of the idea of the body.

41

There also arise purification of the sattva, cheerfulness of the mind, concentration, conquest of the organs, and fitness for the realization of the Self.

Through the practice of cleanliness the sattva material prevails and the mind becomes concentrated and cheerful. The first sign of your becoming religious is that you are cheerful. Gloominess may be a sign of dyspepsia, but it is surely not religion. A pleasurable feeling is the nature of the sattva. Everything is pleasurable to the sāttvika man; and when this comes, know that you are progressing in yoga. All pain is caused by tamas; so you must get rid of it. Moroseness is one of the results of tamas. The strong, the well-knit, the young, the healthy, the daring alone are fit to be yogis. To the yogi everything is bliss, every human face that he sees brings cheerfulness to him. That is the sign of a virtuous man. Misery is caused by sin and by nothing else. What business have you with clouded faces? It is terrible. If you have a clouded face do not go out that day; shut yourself up in your room. What right have you to carry this disease out into the world? When your mind has become controlled you have control over the whole body; instead of being a slave to this machine, you make the machine your slave. Instead of this machine's being able to drag the soul down, it becomes its greatest helpmate.

42

From contentment comes superlative happiness.

43

The mortification of the organs and the body,

through the destruction of their impurities, brings powers to them.

The results of mortification are seen immediately, sometimes in heightened powers of vision, sometimes in the hearing of things at a distance, and so on.

44

By the repetition of the mantra comes the realization of the Chosen Deity.[1]

The higher the being that you want to realize, the harder the practice.

45

Through the sacrificing of all to Iśvara comes samādhi.

By resignation to the Lord, samādhi becomes perfect.

46

Posture is that which is firm and pleasant.

Now comes āsana, posture. Until you acquire a firm posture you cannot practise the breathing and other exercises. Firmness of posture means that you do not feel the body at all. Generally speaking, you will find that as soon as you sit for a few minutes you feel all sorts of bodily disturbances. But when you have gone beyond the idea of a gross, physical body, you will lose all sense of the body. You will feel neither pleasure nor pain. And when you again become aware of it you will feel completely rested. This is the only

[1] That aspect of the Godhead which the aspirant accepts as his Chosen Ideal.

real rest that you can give to the body. When you have succeeded in controlling the body and keeping it firm, your practice will be steady; but while you are disturbed by the body, your nerves become disturbed and you cannot concentrate the mind.

47

Through the lessening of the natural tendency [for activity, caused by identification with the body,] and through meditation on the Infinite, [posture becomes firm and pleasant].

We can make the posture firm by thinking of the Infinite. We cannot actually think of the transcendental Infinite, but we can think of the infinite sky.

48

Posture being conquered, the dualities do not obstruct.

The dualities—good and bad, heat and cold, and all the pairs of opposites—will not then disturb you.

49

Control of the motion of exhalation and inhalation follows after this.

When posture has been conquered, the motion of the prāna is then to be broken—that is to say, stopped —and then controlled. Thus we come to prānā-yāma, the controlling of the vital forces of the body. Prāna is not the breath, though it is usually so translated. It is the sum total of the cosmic energy. It is also the energy that is in each body, and its most apparent manifestation is the motion of the lungs.

This motion is caused by prāna drawing in the breath, and it is what we seek to control by prānāyāma. We begin by controlling the breath as the easiest way of getting control of the prāna.

50

Its modifications are threefold, namely, external, internal, and motionless; they are regulated by place, time, and number; and further, they are either long or short.

There are three kinds of motion in prānāyāma: one by which we draw the breath in, another by which we expel it, and a third by which the breath is held in the lungs or stopped from entering the lungs. These, again, vary according to place and time. "Regulated by place" refers to some particular part of the body where the prāna is to be held. "Regulated by time" refers to how long the prāna should be confined to a certain place; and so we are told how many seconds to keep up one motion and how many seconds another. The result of prānāyāma is udghāta, or the awakening of the Kundalini.

51

The fourth is the restraining of the prāna by directing it either to external or to internal objects.

This is the fourth kind of prānāyāma. The prāna can be directed either inside or outside.

[The above aphorism has also been translated and interpreted in the following manner: "The fourth prānāyāma is that which discards both the external and the internal movement of the prāna."

When the external and the internal breathing, regulated by place, time, and number, etc., as described in the preceding aphorism, have been discarded, there then follows the fourth kind of prāṇā-yāma. It consists in the gradual stopping of the course of both exhalation and inhalation; the difference between the one described in the preceding aphorism and the present one is that in the latter the stopping of exhalation and inhalation is affected by objects and is attained by stages. It is characterized by the absence of all movement of the breath, following upon the complete cessation of inhalation and exhalation. Needless to say, these exercises, like the others in rāja-yoga, should be practised under the guidance of a teacher.]

52

By that, the covering of the light of the chitta is attenuated.

The chitta, by its own nature, is endowed with all knowledge. It is made of sattva particles, but is covered by rajas and tamas particles; and by prāṇā-yāma this covering is removed.

53

The mind becomes fit for dhāranā.

After this covering has been removed we are able to concentrate the mind.

54

Pratyāhāra, or the drawing in of the organs, is effected by their giving up their own objects and taking, as it were, the form of the mind-stuff.

The organs are separate states of the mind-stuff. I see a book: the form is not in the book; it is in the mind. Something is outside which calls that form up; but the real form is in the chitta. The organs identify themselves with, and take the forms of, whatever comes to them. If you can restrain the mind-stuff from taking these forms, the mind will remain calm. This is called pratyāhāra.

55

Thence arises supreme control of the organs.

When the yogi has succeeded in preventing the organs from taking the forms of external objects, and in making them remain one with the mind-stuff, then comes perfect control of the organs. When the organs are perfectly under control, every muscle and nerve will be under control, because the organs are the centres of all sensations and of all actions. These organs are divided into organs of action and organs of sensation. When the organs are controlled, the yogi can control all feeling and doing; the whole of the body comes under his control. Then alone does one begin to feel joy in being born. Then one can truthfully say, "Blessed am I that I was born." When that control of the organs is obtained we feel how wonderful this body really is.

THE POWERS

We have now come to the chapter in which the powers of yoga are described.

1

Dhāranā is the holding of the mind to some particular object.

When the mind holds on to some object, either in the body or outside the body, and keeps itself in that state, it has attained dhāranā, concentration.

2

An unbroken flow of knowledge about that object is dhyāna.

When the mind tries to think of one object, to hold itself to one particular spot, such as the top of the head, or the heart, and succeeds in receiving sensations only through that part of the body, and no other part, it has attained dhāranā; and when the mind succeeds in keeping itself in that state for some time, it has attained dhyāna, meditation.

3

When that (i.e. dhyāna) gives up all forms and reveals only the meaning, it is samādhi.

This comes when in meditation the form or the external part is given up. Suppose I am meditating on a book; I have gradually succeeded in concentrating the mind on it, and then in perceiving only the internal sensations, the meaning, unexpressed in any form. That state of dhyāna is called samādhi.

4

[These] three, [when practised] in regard to one object, constitute samyama.

When a man can direct his mind to any particular object and fix it there, and then keep it there for a long time, separating the object from the internal part, he has attained samyama. In the practice of samyama, dhāranā, dhyāna, and samādhi follow one another and all three are directed to one object. The form of the thing has vanished and only its meaning remains in the mind.

5

Through the attainment of that (i.e. samyama) comes the light of knowledge.

When one has succeeded in practising samyama, all the powers come under one's control. This is the great instrument of the yogi. The objects of knowledge are infinite, and they are divided into gross, grosser, grossest, and fine, finer, finest, and so on. Samyama should be first applied to gross things, and when one begins to get knowledge of the gross, slowly, by stages, it should be applied to finer things.

6

That (i.e. samyama) should be practised in stages.

This is a note of warning not to attempt to go too fast.

7

These three disciplines are more internal than
those that precede.

We have described pratyāhāra, prānāyāma, āsana,
yama, and niyama before; they are more external than
dhāranā, dhyāna, and samādhi. When a man has
attained to these latter he may attain to such powers
as omniscience and omnipotence, but that is not salvation. These three do not make the mind nirvikalpa,
free from modifications, but leave the seeds of future
embodiment. Only when the seeds are, as the yogi
says, fried, do they lose the possibility of producing
further plants. These powers cannot fry the seed.

8

But even they (i.e. dhāranā, dhyāna, and samādhi)
are external to the seedless [samādhi].

Compared with that seedless samādhi, therefore,
even these are external. We have not yet reached the
real samādhi, the highest; we are in a lower stage, in
which the universe still exists as we see it and in which
lie all the powers described in the present chapter.

9

By the suppression of the disturbing impressions
of the mind, and by the rise of impressions of control, the mind which persists in that state of control
is said to attain the controlling modifications.

That is to say, in the first state of samādhi the
modifications of the mind have been controlled, but
not perfectly, because if they were, there would be no
modifications. If there is a modification which impels

the mind to rush out through the senses, and the yogi tries to control it, that very control will be another modification. One wave will be checked by another wave; so it will not be the real samādhi, in which all the waves subside, since the control itself will remain as a wave. Yet this lower samādhi is very much nearer to the higher samādhi than when the mind bubbles up.

10

Its flow becomes steady by habit.

The flow of this continuous control of the mind becomes steady when practised day after day, and the mind obtains the faculty of constant concentration.

11

Taking in all sorts of objects and concentrating upon one object are two modifications of the mind. When the first of these is suppressed and the other manifested, the chitta acquires the modification called samādhi.

The mind generally takes up various objects, runs into all sorts of things. That is the lower state. There is a higher state of the mind, when it takes up one object and excludes all others. The result of this is samādhi.

12

The modification called one-pointedness of the chitta is acquired when the impression that is past and that which is present are similar.

How are we to know that the mind has become concentrated? The idea of time will vanish. The greater the amount of time that passes unnoticed, the more deeply concentrated we are. In everyday life we see that when we are interested in a book we do not note the time at all, and when we leave the book we are often surprised to find how many hours have passed. All time will have a tendency to be unified in the one present. So the definition is given: when the past and present become one, the mind is said to be concentrated.[1]

13

In this way (i.e. by the three modifications mentioned above) is explained the threefold transformation as to form, time, and state in matter and in the organs.

Aphorisms 9, 11, and 12 have explained the threefold transformation in the mind-stuff, or chitta. In like manner are explained the transformations in matter and in the organs. Suppose there is a lump of earth. When it is transformed into a pot, it gives up the form of the lump and takes that of the pot. This is called "transformation as to form." Concerning "transformation as to time," there are three aspects of time: past, present, and future. One can view the pot in any of

[1] The difference between the three kinds of concentration mentioned in aphorisms 9, 11, and 12 is as follows: In the first, the disturbed impressions are merely held back, but not altogether obliterated by the impressions of control, which have just come in; in the second, the former are completely suppressed by the latter, which stand in bold relief; while in the third, which is the highest, there is no question of suppressing, but only similar impressions succeed each other in a stream.

these three aspects. Lastly, the pot may be thought of
as new, old, or as it is going to be. This is called "transformation as to state." Now, referring to aphorisms 9,
11, and 12, the mind-stuff changes into vrittis. This
is transformation as to form. When it passes through
past, present, and future moments of time, it is transformation as to time. And lastly, when the disturbing
impressions of the mind-stuff are strong and the controlling impressions are weak (see aphorism 9), and
vice versa, it is transformation as to state. Since the
mind is an organ, thus is explained transformation of
the organs as to form, time, and state, as mentioned in
the text. The similar transformation of matter has been
explained above. The concentrations taught in the
preceding aphorisms give the yogi a voluntary control
over the transformations of his mind-stuff, which
alone enables him to practise samyama as described
in III. 4. It should be noted that all entities except
the Purusha, or Self, are subject to the threefold transformation mentioned in the text.

14

**That which is acted upon by transformations,
either past, present, or yet to be manifested, is the
substance qualified.**

That is to say, the "substance qualified" is the substance which is being acted upon by time and by the
samskāras, and is always getting changed and being
manifested.

15

**The succession of changes is the cause of mani-
fold evolution.**

16

Through the practice of samyama on the three sorts of changes comes the knowledge of the past and future.

We must not lose sight of the definition of samyama. When the mind has attained to that state in which it identifies itself with the internal impression of the object, leaving the external, and when, by long practice, that impression is retained by the mind, and the mind can get into that state in a moment, that is samyama. If a man in that state wants to know the past and future, he has to practise samyama on the changes in the samskāras (III. 13). Some are working themselves out at present, some have already worked themselves out, and some are waiting to work; so by practising samyama on these he knows the past and future.

17

Through samyama on word, meaning, and knowledge, which are ordinarily confused, comes the knowledge of all animal sounds.

"Word" refers to the external object that stimulates a mental state; "meaning" represents the internal sensation, which travels to the brain through the channels of the indriyas, conveying the external vibration to the mind; and "knowledge" represents the reaction of the mind, with which comes perception. These three, confused, make up our sense-objects. Suppose I hear a word. There is first the external vibration, next the internal sensation carried to the mind by the organ of hearing; then the mind reacts and I know the word. The word I know is a mixture of these three: vibration, sensation, and reaction. Ordinarily they are inseparable; but by practice the yogi can separate them. When a man has attained to this, if he practises samyama on any sound, he understands the meaning which that sound was intended to express, whether it was made by a human being or by any other animal.

18

Through the perceiving of the impressions [comes] the knowledge of past life.

Each experience that we have comes in the form of a wave in the chitta; this subsides and becomes finer and finer, but is never lost. It remains there in a subtle form, and if we can bring this wave up again, it becomes a memory. So if the yogi can practise samyama on these past impressions in the mind, he will begin to remember all his past lives.

19

Through the practice of samyama on the signs on another's body comes knowledge of his mind.

Each man has particular signs on his body, which differentiate him from others. When the yogi practises samyama on the signs peculiar to a certain man, he knows the nature of that man's mind.

20

But not its contents, that not being the object of the samyama.

By practising samyama on the body he would not know the contents of the mind. That would require a twofold samyama: first on the signs on the body and then on the mind itself. The yogi would then know everything in that mind.

21

Through the practice of samyama on the form of the body, the power of perceiving forms being obstructed and the power of manifestation in the eye being separated [from the form], the yogi's body becomes unseen.

A yogi standing in the middle of this room can apparently vanish. He does not really vanish, but he will not be seen by anyone. The form and the body are, as it were, separated. You must remember that this can only be done when the yogi has attained to that power of concentration when the form and the thing formed have been separated. Then he practises samyama on that form, and the power to perceive forms is obstructed, because the power of perceiving forms comes from the junction of the forms and the things formed.

22

In this manner the disappearance or concealment of words which are being spoken, and other such things, are also explained.

23

Karma is of two kinds: some to be fructified soon and some to be fructified later. By practising samyama on these, or on the signs called arishta, portents, the yogis know the exact time of their separation from their bodies.

When a yogi practises samyama on his own karma, upon those impressions in his mind which are now working themselves out and those which are just waiting to work, he knows, by those that are waiting, exactly when his body will fall. He knows when he will die—at what hour, even at what minute. The Hindus think very highly of this knowledge or consciousness of the nearness of death, because it is taught in the Gītā that the thoughts at the moment of departure have great influence in determining the next life.

24

By practising samyama on friendship, mercy, and so forth [I. 33] the yogi excels in these respective qualities.

25

Through samyama on the strength of the elephant, and other creatures, their respective strength comes to the yogi.

When a yogi has attained to samyama and wants strength, he practises samyama on the strength of the elephant and gets it. Infinite energy is at the disposal of everyone, if he only knows how to obtain it. The yogi has discovered the science of obtaining it.

26

Through samyama on the effulgent light [I. 36] comes the knowledge of the fine, the obstructed, and the remote.

When the yogi practises samyama on the effulgent light in the heart, he sees things which are very remote, things, for instance, which are happening in a distant place and which are obstructed by mountain barriers, and also things which are very fine.

27

Through samyama on the sun [comes] knowledge of the world.

28

On the moon, knowledge of the cluster of stars.

29

On the pole-star, knowledge of the motion of the stars.

30

[Through samyama] on the navel circle [comes] knowledge of the constitution of the body.

31

On the hollow of the throat, cessation of hunger.

When a man is very hungry, if he can practise samyama on the hollow of the throat, hunger ceases.

32

On the nerve called the kurma, fixity of the body.

When he is practising disciplines the body is not disturbed.

33

On the light emanating from the top of the head, sight of the siddhas.

The siddhas are beings a little above ghosts. When the yogi concentrates his mind on the top of his head he sees these siddhas. The word *siddhas* does not here refer to those men who have become free, a sense in which it is often used.

34

Or by the power of pratibhā [comes] all knowledge.

All these can come without any samyama to the man who has the power of pratibhā, spontaneous enlightenment through purity. When a man has risen to a high state of pratibhā he has that great light. All things are apparent to him. Everything comes to him naturally without practising samyama.

35

[Through samyama] on the heart [comes] knowledge of minds.

36

Enjoyment comes through the non-discrimination of the Soul and the sattva (buddhi), which are totally different. This enjoyment is for the sake of the Soul. There is another state of the sattva, called svārtha (its own pure state). The practice of samyama on this state gives the knowledge of the Purusha.

The Purusha and the sattva, or buddhi, which is a modification of prakriti, are totally different from each other. But the Purusha is reflected in the buddhi and identifies Itself with the different states of the buddhi, such as happiness or misery, and thus regards Itself as happy or miserable. These experiences of the buddhi are not for its own sake but for that of another, namely, the Soul. But there is another state of the buddhi, which serves its own purpose. In that state it is free from the sense of "me and mine." Devoid of impurities, the buddhi becomes pervaded by the light of the Purusha; it reflects the Purusha alone. Becoming introspective, it is related only to the Purusha and becomes independent of all other relations. When one concentrates on this aspect of the buddhi, one attains the knowledge of the Purusha. The reason for practising samyama on the purified buddhi is that the Purusha Itself can never be the object of knowledge, since It is the knower.

37

From that arises the knowledge of [supernatural] hearing, touching, seeing, tasting, and smelling, which belong to pratibhā.

38

These are obstacles to samādhi, but they are powers in the worldly state.

To the yogi, knowledge of the enjoyments of the world comes by the junction of the Purusha and the mind. If he wants to practise samyama on the knowledge that they are two different things, nature and Self, he gets knowledge of the Purusha. From that arises discrimination. When he has got that discrimination he gets the pratibhā, the light of supreme knowledge. The powers which the yogi obtains, however, are obstructions to the attainment of the highest goal, the knowledge of the Pure Self, or freedom.

These are to be met on the way, and if the yogi rejects them he attains the highest. If he is tempted to acquire these, his farther progress is barred.

39

When the cause of bondage has become loosened, the yogi, by his knowledge of the channels of activity of the chitta (i.e. the nerves), enters another's body.

The yogi can enter a dead body and make it get up and move, even while he himself is working in his own body. Or he can enter a living body and hold that man's mind and organs in check, and for the time being act through the body of that man. This the yogi does by discriminating between the Purusha and nature. If he wants to enter another's body he practises samyama on that body and enters it, because not only is his Self omnipresent, but also his mind, as Yoga teaches. It is one bit of the universal mind. At first, however, it can work only through the nerve currents in his own body. But when the yogi has loosened himself from these nerve currents, his mind can work through other bodies.

40

When he has conquered the current called the udāna, the yogi does not sink in water or in swamps, he can walk on thorns and so forth, and can die at will.

The udāna is the nerve current that governs the lungs and all the upper parts of the body, and when the yogi has mastered it he becomes light in weight. He does not sink in water, he can walk on thorns and sword blades and stand in fire, and can depart from this life whenever he likes.

41

Through the conquest of the current called the samāna he is surrounded by a blaze of light.

Whenever he wishes, light flashes from his body.

42

Through samyama on the relation between the ear and ākāśa comes divine hearing.

There is ākāśa, ether, and there is also the instrument, the ear. By practising samyama on them the yogi gets supernormal hearing; he hears anything he wants to. He can hear sounds uttered miles away.

43

By practising samyama on the relation between ākāśa and the body and regarding himself to be as light as cotton-wool, and so forth, the yogi can go through the skies.

Ākāśa is the material of this body; the body is only ākāśa in a certain form. If the yogi practises samyama on this material of his body, it acquires the lightness of ākāśa and he can go anywhere through the air.

44

Through samyama on the real modifications of the mind, outside the body, called great disembodiedness, comes disappearance of the covering to light.

The mind in its foolishness thinks that it is working in one body. Why should I be bound by one system of nerves and limit the ego to only one body, if the mind is omnipresent? There is no reason why I should. The yogi wants to feel the ego wherever he likes. The mental waves which arise in the absence of egoity in the body are called "real modifications" or "great disembodiedness." When he has succeeded in practising samyama on these modifications, all the covering to light goes away and all darkness and ignorance vanish. Everything appears to him to be full of consciousness.

45

Through samyama on the gross and fine forms of the elements, their essential traits, the inherence of the gunas in them, and their contributing to the experience of the Soul comes mastery of the elements.

The yogi practises samyama on the elements, first on the gross and then on the fine. This samyama is taken up mostly by a sect of Buddhists. They take a lump of clay and practise samyama on that, and gradually they begin to see the fine materials of which it is composed; and when they have known all the fine materials in it, they get power over those elements. So with all the elements. The yogi can conquer them all.

46

From that come minuteness and the rest of the powers, glorification of the body, and indestructibility of the bodily qualities.

This means that the yogi has attained the eight supernatural powers. He can make himself as minute as an atom or as huge as a mountain, as heavy as the earth or as light as air; he can reach anything he likes, he can rule everything he wants, he can conquer everything he wants, and so on. A lion sits at his feet like a lamb, and all his desires are fulfilled at will.

47

"Glorification of the body" means beauty, complexion, strength, adamantine hardness.

The body becomes indestructible. Nothing can injure it. Nothing can destroy it until the yogi wishes. "Breaking the rod of time, he lives in this universe in his body." In the Vedas it is written that for such a man there is no more disease, death, or pain.

48

Through samyama on the perception, by the organs, of external objects, the knowledge that follows, the "I-consciousness" that accompanies this knowledge, the inherence of the gunas in all of these, and their contributing to the experience of the Soul comes the conquest of the organs.

In the perception of external objects the organs leave their places in the mind and go towards the objects; this process is followed by knowledge. Ego also is present in the act. When the yogi practises samyama on these and the other two, by gradation, he conquers the organs. Take up anything that you see or feel—a book, for instance: first concentrate the mind on it, then on the knowledge that is in the form of a book, and then on the ego that sees the book, and so on. By this practice all the organs will be conquered.

49

From that come to the body the power of **rapid movement** like that of the mind, power of the **organs independent of the body**, and the **conquest of nature**.

Just as by the conquest of the elements comes a glorified body, so from the conquest of the organs come the above-mentioned powers.

50

Through samyama on the discrimination between the sattva and the Purusha come omnipotence and omniscience.

When nature has been conquered, and the difference between the Purusha and nature realized—that the Purusha is indestructible, pure, and perfect, and nature, Its opposite—then come omnipotence and omniscience.

51

Through the giving up of even these powers comes the destruction of the very seed of evil, and this leads to kaivalya (isolation).

The yogi attains aloneness and becomes free. When one gives up even the ideas of omnipotence and omniscience, there comes the entire rejection of enjoyment, of the temptations from celestial beings. When the yogi has seen all these wonderful powers and rejected them, he reaches the goal. What are all these powers? Simply manifestations. They are no better than dreams. Even omnipotence is a dream. It depends on the mind. So long as there is a mind it can be omnipotent; but the goal is beyond even the mind.

52

The yogi should not feel allured or flattered by the overtures of celestial beings, for fear of evil again.

There are other dangers too: gods and other beings come to tempt the yogi. They do not want anyone to be perfectly free. They are jealous, just as we are, and are even worse than us sometimes. They are very much afraid of losing their positions. Those yogis who do not reach perfection become gods after death; leaving the direct road, they go into one of the side-streets and get these powers. Then they have to be born again. But he who is strong enough to withstand these temptations, and goes straight to the goal, becomes free.

53

Through samyama on a particle of time and that which precedes and succeeds it comes discrimination.

How are we to avoid all these things—these devas and heavens and powers? By discrimination, by knowing good from evil. Therefore a samyama is prescribed by which the power of discrimination can be strengthened. This is done through samyama on a particle of time and the time preceding and following it.

54

Those things which cannot be differentiated by species, sign, or place—even they will be differentiated by the above samyama.

The misery we suffer from is the result of ignorance,

of non-discrimination between the real and the unreal.
We all take the bad for the good, the dream for the
reality. The Self is the only reality, and we have forgotten It. The body is an unreal dream, and we all
think we are bodies. This non-discrimination is the
cause of misery. It is caused by ignorance. When discrimination comes it brings strength. Then alone can
we avoid all these various ideas of body, heavens, and
gods. We differentiate between objects by means of
species, sign, and place. For instance, take a cow. The
cow is differentiated from the dog by species. Even
with cows alone, how do we make the distinction between one cow and another? By signs. If two objects
are exactly similar, they can be distinguished if they
are in different places. When objects are so mixed up
that even these differentiae will not help us, the
power of discrimination acquired by the above-mentioned practice will give us the ability to distinguish
them. The highest philosophy of the yogi is based
upon this fact: that the Purusha is pure and perfect
and is the only simple substance that exists in this
universe. The body and mind are compounds, and yet
we are for ever identifying ourselves with them. This
is the great mistake—that the distinction has been
lost. When the power of discrimination has been
attained, a man sees that everything in this world,
mental and physical, is a compound, and, as such,
cannot be the Purusha.

55

The saving knowledge is that knowledge of discrimination which simultaneously covers all objects
in all their variations.

This knowledge is called "saving" because it takes the yogi across the ocean of birth and death. The whole of prakriti in all its states, subtle and gross, is within the grasp of this knowledge. There is no succession in perception of this knowledge; it takes in all things simultaneously, at a glance.

56

By the similarity of purity between the sattva and the Purusha comes kaivalya.

When the Purusha realizes that It depends on nothing in the universe, from the gods to the lowest atom, It attains the state of kaivalya, or perfection. Kaivalya is the goal. When the Self attains this state, It realizes that It has always been alone and "isolated," and that It did not require anything to make It happy. As long as we want somebody or something else for our happiness, so long we are slaves. When the Purusha knows that freedom is Its very nature and that It does not need anything to attain perfection, when It knows that nature is transitory and really meaningless, that very moment the Purusha attains liberation and becomes "isolated" from nature. This state is attained when the mixture of purity and impurity called the sattva, that is to say, the intellect, has been made as pure as the Purusha Itself; then the sattva reflects only the unqualified essence of purity, which is the Purusha.

INDEPENDENCE

1

The siddhis, or powers, are attained through birth, chemical means, the power of words, mortification, or concentration.

Sometimes a man is born with the siddhis, or powers; of course these he had earned in his previous incarnation. This time he is born, as it were, to enjoy their fruits. It is said of Kapila, the great father of the Sāmkhya philosophy, that he was a born siddha, which means, literally, a man who has attained to success.

The yogis claim that these powers can also be gained by chemical means. All of you know that chemistry originally began as alchemy; men began to search for the philosophers' stone and elixirs of life, and so forth. In India there was a sect called the Rasāyanas. According to them, subtle theories, knowledge, spirituality, and religion were all very good, but the body was the only instrument by which to attain results. If the body came to an end every now and again, it would take so much more time to attain the goal. For instance, a man wants to practise yoga or wants to become spiritual. Before he has advanced very far he dies. Then he takes another body and begins again, then dies, and so on. In this way much time is lost in dying and being born again. If the body could be made strong and perfect, so that it could free itself from birth and death, we should have so much more time to become spiritual.

So these Rasāyanas said that we should first make the body very strong. They claimed that this body could be made immortal. Their idea was that if the mind manufactured the body, and if it was true that each mind is only one outlet of the infinite energy, there should be no limit to each outlet's getting power from outside. Therefore why should it be impossible to keep our bodies alive all the time? We have to manufacture all the bodies that we ever have. As soon as this body dies we shall have to manufacture another. If we can do that, why cannot we do it just here and now, without getting out of the present body? The theory is perfectly correct. If it is possible for us to live after death and make other bodies, why is it impossible for us to make bodies here, without entirely dissolving this body—simply changing it continually? They also thought that in mercury and sulphur was hidden a most wonderful power, and that by certain preparations of these a man could keep the body alive as long as he liked. Others believed that certain drugs could bring powers, such as flying through the air. Many of the most wonderful medicines of the present day we owe to the Rasāyanas, notably the use of metals in medicine. Certain sects of yogis claim that many of their principal teachers are still living in their old bodies. Patanjali, the great authority on Yoga, does not deny this.

The power of words: There are certain sacred

words, called mantras, which, when repeated under proper conditions, are able to produce these extraordinary powers. We are living in the midst of such a mass of miracles, day and night, that we do not think anything of them. There is no limit to man's power: the power of words and the power of mind.

Mortification: You find that every religion prescribes such disciplines as mortification and asceticism. In matters like these the Hindus always go to extremes. You will find men holding their hands up all their lives, until their hands wither and die. Men keep standing, day and night, until their feet swell, and if they live, the legs become so stiff in this position that they can no more bend them, but have to stand all their lives. I once saw a man who had kept his hands raised in this way, and I asked him how he felt when he did it first. He said it was awful torture. It was such torture that he had to go to a river and put himself in water, and that allayed the pain for a little while. After a month he did not suffer much. Through such practices the powers, or siddhis, can be attained.

Concentration: This is yoga proper; this is the principal theme of this science, and it is the highest discipline. The preceding ones are only secondary, and we cannot attain to the goal through them. Samādhi is the means through which we can gain anything and everything—mental, moral, and spiritual.

2

The change into another species is effected by the filling in of nature.

Patanjali has advanced the proposition that these powers come by birth or by chemical means or through mortification. He also has said that the body can be kept alive for any length of time. Now he goes on to state what is the cause of the change of the body into another species. He says that this is done by the filling in of nature, which he explains in the next aphorism.

3

Good and bad deeds are not the direct causes of the transformations of nature, but they act as breakers of obstacles to its evolutions—as a farmer breaks the obstacles to the course of water, which then flows down by its own nature.

The water for irrigating the fields is already in the canal, only held back by gates. The farmer opens these gates and the water flows in by itself, by the law of gravitation. So all progress and power are already in man. Perfection is man's very nature; only it is barred off and so prevented from taking its proper course. If anyone can take the bar away, in rushes nature. Then the man attains the powers which are his already. Those whom we call wicked become saints as soon as the bar is broken and nature rushes in. It is nature that is driving us towards perfection, and eventually it will bring everyone there. All these practices and struggles to become religious are only negative work, to take off the bars and open the doors to that perfection which is our birthright, our nature.

Today the evolution theory of the ancient yogis will be better understood in the light of modern research. But the theory of the yogis is **a better explanation.**

The two causes of evolution advanced by the moderns, namely, sexual selection and the survival of the fittest, are inadequate. Suppose human knowledge has advanced so much that it has eliminated competition as a factor in the acquiring both of physical sustenance and of a mate; then, according to the moderns, human progress will stop and the race will die. The result of this theory is to furnish every oppressor with an argument to calm the qualms of conscience. Men are not lacking who, posing as philosophers, would kill out all weak and incompetent persons—they are, of course, the only judges of competency—and thus preserve the human race. But the great ancient evolutionist Patanjali declares that the true goal of evolution is the manifestation of the perfection which is already in every being; that this perfection has been barred off, and the infinite tide is struggling to express itself. All this struggle and competition is but the result of our ignorance, because we do not know the proper way to unlock the gate and let the water in. This infinite tide behind must express itself; it is the cause of all manifestation. Competition for survival or sex-gratification is only a momentary, unnecessary, extraneous factor caused by ignorance. Even when all competition has ceased, this perfect nature in us will make us go forward until everyone has attained perfection. Therefore there is no reason to believe that competition is necessary to progress. In the animal the man was suppressed, but as soon as the door was opened, out rushed man. So, too, in man there is the potential god, kept in by the locks and bars of ignorance. When knowledge breaks these bars the god becomes manifest.

4

A yogi can create many minds from his egoity.

The theory of karma is that we experience the results of our good or bad deeds, and the whole scope of philosophy is to help us realize the glory of man. All the scriptures sing the glory of man, of the Soul, and then, in the same breath, they preach karma. A good deed brings one result, and a bad deed another. But if the Soul can be acted upon by a good or bad deed, It amounts to nothing. Bad deeds simply put a bar to the manifestation of the nature of the Purusha; good deeds take the obstacles off, and the glory of the Purusha becomes manifest. The Purusha Itself is never changed. Whatever you do never destroys your own glory, your own nature, because the Soul cannot be acted upon by anything; only a veil is spread before It, hiding Its perfection.

With a view to exhausting their karma quickly, yogis create kāya-vyuha, or groups of bodies, in which to work it out. For all these bodies they create minds from egoity. These are called "created minds" in contradistinction to their original minds.

5

Though the activities of the different created minds are various, the one original mind is the controller of them all.

These different minds, which act in the different bodies, are called "created minds," and the bodies, "created bodies"—that is, manufactured bodies and minds. Matter and mind are like two inexhaustible

storehouses. When you become a yogi you learn the
secret of their control. It was yours all the time, but
you had forgotten it. When you become a yogi you
recollect it. Then you can do anything with it,
manipulate it in any way you like. The material out
of which a created mind is made is the very same material which is used for the macrocosm. It is not that
mind is one thing and matter another; they are different aspects of the same thing. Asmitā, egoity, is the
material, the fine state of existence, out of which these
"created minds" and "created bodies" of the yogi are
manufactured. Therefore when the yogi has found the
secret of these energies of nature, he can manufacture
any number of bodies or minds out of the substance
known as egoity.

6

**Among the various minds, that which is attained
by samādhi is desireless.**

Among all the various minds that we see in various
men, that mind which has attained to samādhi, perfect
concentration, is the highest. A man who has attained
certain powers through medicines, or through mantras,
or through mortifications, still has desires; but he who
has attained to samādhi through concentration is free
from all desires.

7

**Works are neither black nor white for the yogis;
for others they are threefold: black, white, and
mixed.**

When the yogi has attained perfection, his actions,
and the results produced by those actions, do not bind

him, because he is free from desire. He just works on. He works to do good, and he does good; but he does not care for the results, and they will not come to him. But for ordinary men, who have not attained to that highest state, works are of three kinds: black, or evil, white, or good, and mixed.

8

From these threefold works are manifested in each state only those desires [which are] fitting to that state alone. [The others are held in abeyance for the time being.]

Suppose that I have performed the three kinds of karma—good, bad, and mixed—and suppose that I die and become a god in heaven. The desires in a god body are not the same as the desires in a human body. The god body neither eats nor drinks. What becomes of my past unfulfilled karmas, which should produce as their effect the desire to eat and drink? Where do these karmas go when I become a god? The answer is that desires can only manifest themselves in proper environments. Only those desires become active for which the environment is fitted; the rest will remain stored up. In this life we have many godly desires, many human desires, many animal desires. If I take a god body, only the good desires will function, because for them the environment is suitable. And if I take an animal body, only the animal desires will become active, and the good desires will wait. What does this show? It shows that by means of environment we can check desires. Only that karma which is suited to and fitted for the environment will come out. This shows that the power of environment is a great check to control even karma itself.

9

There is consecutiveness in desires, even though separated by species, space, and time, there being identification of memory and impressions.

Experiences becoming fine become impressions; impressions revivified become memory. The word *memory* here includes unconscious co-ordination of past experiences, reduced to impressions, with present conscious action. In each body, only the group of impressions acquired in a similar body becomes the cause of action in that body. The experiences of a dissimilar body are held in abeyance. Each body acts as if it were the descendant of a series of bodies of that species only; thus consecutiveness of desires is not broken.

10

Thirst for happiness being eternal, desires are without beginning.

All experience is preceded by desire for happiness. There is no beginning of experience, since each fresh experience is built upon the tendency generated by past experience; therefore desire is without beginning.

11

[Desire] being held together by cause, effect, support, and objects, in the absence of these it is absent.

Desires are held together by cause and effect;[1] if a

[1] The causes are the "pain-bearing obstructions" (II. 3) and works (IV. 7), and the effects are "species, longevity, and experience of pleasure and pain" (II. 13).

desire has been raised, it does not die without producing its effect. Then again, the mind-stuff is the great storehouse, the receptacle of all past desires reduced to samskāra form; until they have worked themselves out they will not die. Moreover, so long as the senses receive external objects, fresh desires will arise. If it is possible to get rid of the cause, effect, support, and objects of desire, then alone will desires vanish.

12

The past and future exist in their own nature, their difference being due to the differences in the gunas.

The idea is that existence never comes out of non-existence. The past and future, though not existing in a manifested form, exist in a fine form.

13

They are manifested or fine, the gunas being their inmost nature.

The gunas are the three substances—sattva, rajas, and tamas—whose gross state is the tangible universe. Past and future arise from the different modes of manifestation of these gunas.

14

The unity in things follows from the unity in changes [of the gunas].

Though there are three substances, their changes being co-ordinated, all objects manifest a unity.

15

Since perception and desire vary with regard to the same object, mind and object are of different nature.

That is, there is an objective world independent of our minds. This is a refutation of Buddhist idealism. Since different people look at the same thing differently, it cannot be a mere imagination of any particular individual.[2]

16

Things are known or unknown to the mind, being dependent on the colouring which they give to the mind.

17

The states of the mind are always known, because the Lord of the mind, the Purusha, is unchangeable.

The whole gist of this theory is that the universe is both mental and material. Both matter and mind are in a state of flux. What is this book? It is a combination of molecules in constant change: one lot is going out, and another coming in. It is like a whirlpool. But what makes the unity? What makes it the same book? The changes are rhythmical; in harmonious order they are sending impressions to my mind, and these pieced together make a continuous picture, although the parts are continuously changing. The

[2] There is an additional aphorism here in some editions: "The object cannot be said to be dependent on a single mind. There being no proof of its existence, [if the mind did not perceive it,] it would then become non-existent." If the perception of an object were the only criterion of its existence, then, when a man's mind was absorbed in something or was in samādhi, that object would not be perceived by anybody and might as well be said to be non-existent. This is an undesirable conclusion.

mind, too, is continuously changing. Mind and body are like two layers in the same substance, moving at different rates of speed. One being slower and the other quicker, we can distinguish between the two motions. For instance, a train is in motion and a carriage is moving alongside of it. It is possible to determine the motion of both of them, to a certain extent. But still something else is necessary. Motion can only be perceived when there is something else which is not moving. But when two or three things are moving relative to one another, we first perceive the motion of the faster one, and then that of the slower ones. How can the mind perceive? It too is in a flux. Hence another thing is necessary which moves more slowly; then you must think of something in which the motion is still slower, and so on; and you will find no end. Therefore logic compels you to stop somewhere. You must complete the series by knowing something which never changes. Behind this never-ending chain of motion is the Purusha, changeless, colourless, pure. All these impressions are merely reflected upon It, as a magic lantern throws images upon a screen without in any way staining it.

18

The mind is not self-luminous, being an object.

Tremendous power is manifested everywhere by the mind, but it is not self-luminous, not essentially intelligent. The Purusha alone is self-luminous, and It gives Its light to everything. It is the power of the Purusha that is percolating through all matter and energy.

19

On account of its being unable to cognize both at the same time, [the mind is not self-luminous].

If the mind were self-luminous it would be able to cognize itself and its objects at the same time, which it cannot. When it cognizes objects it cannot reflect on itself. Therefore the Purusha is self-luminous and the mind is not.

20

Another cognizing mind being assumed, there will be no end to such assumptions, and confusion of memory will be the result.

Let us suppose that there is another mind which cognizes the ordinary mind; there will then have to be still another to cognize the former, and so there will be no end to it. The result will be confusion of memory; there will be no storehouse of memory.

21

The Essence of Knowledge (the Purusha) is unchangeable; when the mind takes Its form, it becomes conscious.

Patanjali says this to make it more clear that knowledge is not a quality of the Purusha. When the mind comes near the Purusha, the latter is reflected, as it were, upon the mind, and the mind, for the time being, becomes knowing and seems as if it were itself the Purusha.

22

Coloured by the Seer and the seen, the mind is able to understand everything.

On one side of the mind the external world, the seen, is being reflected, and on the other, the Seer is being reflected; thus comes to the mind the power of knowing everything.

23

The mind, though variegated on account of innumerable desires, acts for another (i.e. the Purusha), because it acts in combination.

The mind is a compound of various things and therefore cannot work for itself. Everything that is a combination in this world serves the purpose of another entity for which that combination has been made. So this combination of the mind is for the Purusha.

24

For the discriminating the perception of the mind as Ātman ceases.

Through discrimination the yogi knows that the Purusha is not the mind.

25

Then, bent on discriminating, the mind attains the state preliminary to kaivalya, isolation.

[There is another reading: "Then the mind becomes deep in discrimination and gravitates towards kaivalya."]

Thus the practice of yoga leads to the power of discriminating, to clearness of vision. The veil drops from the eyes and we see things as they are. We find that nature is a compound and is showing its panorama for the satisfaction of the Purusha, who is the witness;

that nature is not the Lord, that all the combinations of nature are simply for the sake of showing these phenomena to the Purusha, the enthroned King within. When discrimination comes by long practice, fear ceases and the mind attains isolation.

26

The thoughts that arise [from time to time] as obstructions to that come from impressions.

All the various ideas that arise, making us believe that we require something external to make us happy, are obstructions to that perfection. The Purusha is happiness and blessedness by Its own nature. But that knowledge is covered over by past impressions. These impressions have to work themselves out.

27

Their destruction is in the same manner as that of ignorance, egoity, and so forth, as said before (II. 10).

28

Even when arriving at the right discriminative knowledge of the essences, he who gives up its fruits —unto him comes, as the result of perfect discrimination, the samādhi called the "cloud of virtue."

When the yogi has attained to discrimination, all the powers mentioned in the last chapter come to him; but the true yogi rejects them all. Unto him comes a peculiar knowledge, a particular light, called the dharmamegha, the "cloud of virtue." All the great prophets of the world whom history has recorded had this. They had found the whole foundation of knowledge within themselves. Truth to them had become real. Peace and calmness and perfect purity became their own nature after they had given up the vanities of powers.

29

From that comes the cessation of pain and works.

When that "cloud of virtue" has come, then no more is there fear of falling; nothing can drag the yogi down. No more will there be evil for him; no more will there be pain.

30

Then knowledge, bereft of covering and impurities, becomes infinite and the knowable becomes small.

Knowledge itself is there; its covering is gone. One of the Buddhist scriptures defines the Buddha—which is the name of a state—as infinite knowledge, infinite as the sky. Jesus attained to that and became the Christ. All of you will attain to that state. Knowledge becoming infinite, the knowable becomes small. The whole universe, with all its objects of knowledge, becomes as nothing before the Purusha. The ordinary man thinks himself very small, because to him the knowable seems to be infinite.

31

Then are finished the successive transformations of the gunas, they having attained their end.

Then all these various transformations of the gunas, which change from species to species, cease for ever.

32

The changes that exist in relation to moments, and which are perceived at the other end (i.e. at the end of a series), are what is meant by succession.

Patanjali here defines the word *succession*: the changes that exist in relation to moments. While I think, many moments pass, and with each moment there is a change of idea; but I only perceive these changes at the end of a series. This is called succession. But for the mind that has realized omnipresence there is no succession. Everything has become present for it. To it the present alone exists; the past and future are lost. Time stands controlled; all knowledge is there in one second. Everything is known in a flash.

33

The resolution of the gunas in the inverse order, when they are bereft of any motive of action for the Purusha, is kaivalya (isolation or freedom); or kaivalya is the establishment of the Power of Knowledge in Its own nature.

Nature's task is done, this unselfish task which our sweet nurse, nature, has imposed upon herself. She gently takes the self-forgetting soul by the hand, as it were, and shows it all the experiences in the universe, all manifestations, bringing it higher and higher through various bodies, till its lost glory comes back and it remembers its own nature. Then the kind mother goes back the same way she came, for others who also have lost their way in the trackless desert of life. Thus is she working, without beginning and without end; and thus, through pleasure and pain, through good and evil, the infinite river of souls is flowing into the ocean of perfection, of Self-realization.

Glory unto those who have realized their own nature! May their blessings be on us all!

APPENDIX

APPENDIX

REFERENCES TO YOGA

Śvetāśvatara Upanishad

Chapter II

6

Where the fire is kindled by rubbing, where the air is controlled, where the soma flows over, there a [perfect] mind is created.

8

Placing the body in a straight posture, with the chest, the neck, and the head held erect, making the organs and the mind enter the heart, the sage crosses all the fearful currents by means of the raft of Brahman.

9

The man of well regulated endeavours controls the prāna, and when it has become quieted, breathes out through the nostrils. The wise man undistractedly holds his mind, as a charioteer restrains restive horses.

10

In [lonely] places, such as mountain caves, where the floor is even, free from pebbles or sand, free from fire, where there are no disturbing noises from men or waterfalls, in places pleasing to the mind and not painful to the eyes, yoga is to be practised.

11

When yoga is practised, the forms which appear first and which gradually manifest Brahman are those of snowflakes, smoke, sun, wind, fire, fire-flies, lightning, crystal, and the moon.

12

When the perceptions of smell, taste, touch, form, and sound, arising from earth, water, air, fire, and ākāśa, as described in yoga, have taken place, then yoga has begun. Unto him disease does not come, nor old age nor death, who has got a body purified by the fire of yoga.

13

The first signs of entering yoga are lightness, health, absence of desire, a good complexion, a beautiful voice, an agreeable odour of the body, and slight excretions.

14

As a lump of gold or silver covered with earth shines brightly when well cleaned, so the embodied man, realizing the truth of Ātman, attains Non-duality and becomes sorrowless and blessed.

Yājnavalkya, Quoted by Śankara

"After practising the postures as desired, according to the rules, O Gārgi, a man who has conquered the postures will practise prānāyāma.

"Seated in an easy posture, on a [deer or tiger] skin placed on kuśa grass, worshipping Ganapati with fruits and sweetmeats, placing the right palm on the left, holding the neck and head in the same line, the lips closed and firm, facing the east or the north, the eyes fixed on the tip of the nose, avoiding too much food or fasting, the nādis should be purified, without which the practice will be fruitless. Thinking of [the seed-word] *Hum,* at the junction of the Pingalā and the Idā (the right and the left nostrils), the Idā should be filled with external air in twelve seconds; then the yogi meditates on fire in the same place, with the word *Rung,* and while meditating thus, slowly ejects the air through the Pingalā. Again filling in, through the Pingalā, the air should be slowly ejected through the Idā in the same way. This should be practised for three or four years, or three or four months, according to the directions of a guru, in secret (alone in a room), in the early morning, at midday, in the evening, and at midnight [until] the nerves become purified. Lightness of body, clear complexion, good appetite, and hearing of the Nāda are the signs of the purification of the nerves. Then should be practised prānāyāma, composed of rechaka (exhalation), kumbhaka (retention), and puraka (inhalation). Joining the prāna with the apāna is prānāyāma.

"After filling the body from the head to the feet in sixteen seconds, the prāna is to be expelled in thirty-two seconds, and for sixty-four, kumbhaka should be practised.

"There is another prānāyāma, in which kumbhaka should first be made for sixty-four seconds, then the prāna should be expelled in sixteen, and the body next filled in sixteen seconds.

"By prānāyāma the impurities of the body are expelled; by dhāranā, the impurities of the mind; by pratyāhāra, the impurities of attachment; and by samādhi is taken off everything that hides the lordship of the Soul."

Sāmkhya Philosophy

Book III

29

Through intensity of meditation there come to the Purusha all the powers of nature.

30

Meditation is the destruction of attachment.

31

It is perfected by the suppression of the modifications.

32

It is perfected by dhāranā, posture, and performance of one's duties.

33

Restraint of the prāna is effected by means of expulsion and retention.

34

Posture is that which is steady and easy.

36

Meditation is also perfected by non-attachment and practice.

74

By reflection on the principles of nature and by giving them up as "not this, not this," discrimination is perfected.

Book IV

3

The student should repeatedly hear instruction [from the scriptures and the teacher].

5

As the hawk becomes unhappy if his food is taken away from him and happy if he gives it up himself, [so he who gives up everything voluntarily is happy].

6

As the snake is happy in giving up his old skin, [so he who gives up everything voluntarily is happy].

8

That which is not a means of liberation is not to be thought of; it becomes a cause of bondage, as in the case of Bharata.[1]

[1] According to the story, King Bharata on his death-bed brooded over his pet deer and consequently was reborn as a deer.

9

Association with many persons creates passion, aversion, and so forth, and is an obstruction to meditation, as with the shell bracelets on the virgin's hand.[2]

10

It is the same even with two [persons].

11

The renouncers of hope are happy, like the girl Pingalā.[3]

13

Though an aspirant should show devotion to many scriptures and teachers, he must take from all of them the essence only, as a bee takes the essence from many flowers.

14

One whose mind has become concentrated like an arrow-maker's is not disturbed in his samādhi.

15

As great harm is done in a worldly undertaking

[2] A maiden, who wore a number of bracelets on her wrists, was massaging her father in order to put him to sleep. But the friction of the bracelets made a noise, disturbing his rest.

[3] The prostitute Pingalā, eagerly awaiting the arrival of her paramour, felt extremely unhappy because he did not come. Suddenly giving up all thought of him, she went to her room and spent the night free from anxiety.

when the prescribed rules are violated, so it is also with meditation.

19

Through continence, reverence, and devotion to the guru, success is attained after a long time [as in the case of Indra].

20

There is no law as to time, as in the case of Vāmadeva.[4]

24

Or [success is attained] through association with one who has attained perfection.

27

As the sage Sauvari [who practised yoga for a long time] could not appease his desires through enjoyments, so it is also with others.

Book V

128

As recovery through medicines, and so forth, cannot be denied, so neither can the siddhis attained through yoga.

Book VI

Any posture which is easy and steady is an āsana; there is no injunction [about any particular posture].

[4] It is said that Vāmadeva attained Knowledge while still in his mother's womb.

Vyāsa Sutras

Chapter IV, Section i

7

Worship is possible in a sitting posture. [Therefore one should be seated while worshipping.]

8

Because of meditation.[5]

9

Because the meditating [person] is compared to the immovable earth.

10

Also because the Smritis say so.

11

There is no law of place [for meditation]; wherever the mind is concentrated, meditation should be practised.

These several extracts give an idea of what other systems of Indian philosophy have to say about Yoga.

[5] When we see a man seated without moving his limbs, we say that he is meditating. Therefore meditation is possible for a person who is seated.

MISCELLANEOUS

THE POWERS OF THE MIND

(Delivered at Los Angeles, January 8, 1900)

ALL OVER THE WORLD there has been a belief in the supernatural, throughout the ages. All of us have heard of extraordinary happenings, and many of us have had some personal experience of them. I should like to introduce the subject by telling you certain facts which have come within my own experience.

I once heard of a man who, if anyone went to him with questions in his mind, would answer them immediately; and I was also informed that he foretold events. I was curious and went to see him with a few friends. Each one of us had something in his mind to ask; and to avoid mistakes, each of us wrote down his question and put it in his pocket. As soon as the man saw us, he repeated our questions and gave the answers to them. Then he wrote something on a piece of paper, which he folded up and asked me to sign on the back, and said: "Don't look at it; put it in your pocket. This will be your next question; and here is the answer." And so to each one of us. He next told us about some events that would happen to us in the future. Then he said, "Now think of a word or a sentence from any language you like." I thought of a long sentence from Sanskrit, a language of which he was entirely ignorant. "Now take out the paper from

233

your pocket," he said. The Sanskrit sentence was written there! He had written it an hour before, with the remark, "In confirmation of what I have written, this man will think of this sentence." It was correct. Another of us who had been given a similar paper, which he had signed and placed in his pocket, was also asked to think of a sentence. He thought of a sentence in Arabic, which it was still less possible for the man to know; it was some passage from the Koran. And my friend found this written down on the paper. Another of us was a physician. He thought of a sentence from a German medical book. It was written on his paper.

Several days later I went to this man again, thinking possibly I had been deluded somehow before. I took other friends, and on this occasion also he came out wonderfully triumphant.

Another time, I was in the city of Hyderabad in India, and I was told of a brāhmin there who could produce numbers of things from nobody knew where. This man was in business there; he was a respectable gentleman. And I asked him to show me his tricks. It so happened that this man had fever; and in India there is a general belief that if a holy man puts his hand on a sick man he will be well. This brāhmin came to me and said, "Sir, put your hand on my head, so that my fever may be cured." I said, "Very good; but you show me your tricks." He promised. I put my hand on his head as desired, and later he came to fulfil his promise. He had only a strip of cloth about his loins; we took everything else off him. I had a blanket, which I gave him to wrap round himself because it was cold, and made him sit in a corner. Twenty-five pairs of eyes were looking at him. And he said, "Now look here; write down anything you want." We all wrote down names of fruits that never grew in that locality—bunches of grapes, oranges, and so on. And we gave him those bits of paper. And there came from under his blanket bushels of grapes, oranges, and so on—so much that if all that fruit had been weighed it would have been twice as heavy as the man. He asked us to eat the fruit. Some of us objected, thinking it was hypnotism; but the man himself began eating; so we all ate. It was all right.

He ended by producing a mass of roses. Each flower was perfect, with dew-drops on the petals, not one crushed, not one injured. And masses of them! When I asked the man for an explanation, he said, "It is all sleight-of-hand."

Whatever it was, it seemed to be impossible that it could be sleight-of-hand merely. Where could he have got such large quantities of things?

Well, I have seen many things like that. Going about India, you find hundreds of similar things in different places. These happen in every country. Even in this country you will find some such wonderful things. Of course there is a great deal of fraud, no doubt; but then, whenever you see fraud, you have also to say that that fraud is an imitation. There must be some truth somewhere that is being imitated; you cannot imitate nothing. Imitation must be of something substantially true.

In very remote times in India, thousands of years ago, these things used to happen even more than they do today. It seems to me that when a country becomes very thickly populated, psychical power deteriorates. Given a vast country, thinly inhabited, there will perhaps be more of psychical power there. These facts the Hindus, being analytically minded, took up and investigated. And they came to certain remarkable conclusions; that is, they made a science of them. They found out that all these happenings, though extraordinary, are also natural; there is nothing supernatural about them. They are under laws just as any other physical phenomena are. It is not a freak of nature that a man is born with such powers. They can be systematically studied and acquired. This science they call the science of Rāja-yoga. There are thousands of people who practise it.

The conclusion of Rāja-yoga is that all these extraordinary powers are in the mind of man. This mind is a part of the universal mind. Each mind is connected with every other mind; and each mind, wherever it is located, is in actual communication with the whole world.

Have you ever noticed the phenomenon that is called thought-transference? A man here is thinking something and that thought is manifested in somebody else, in some other place. With preparations—not by chance—a man wants to send a thought to another mind at a distance, and this other mind knows that a thought is coming, and he receives it exactly as it is sent out. Distance makes no difference. The thought goes and reaches the other man, and he understands it. If your mind were an isolated something here, and my mind were an isolated something there, and there were no connexion between the two, how would it be possible for my thought to reach you? In ordinary cases it is not my thought that is reaching you direct; but my thought has got to be dissolved into ethereal vibrations, and those ethereal vibrations go into your brain, and they have to be resolved again into your own thoughts. Here is a dissolution of thought, and there is a resolution of thought. It is a roundabout process. But in telepathy there is no such thing; it is direct.

This shows that there is a continuity of mind, as the yogis call it. The mind is universal. Your mind, my mind, all these little minds, are fragments of that universal mind, little waves in the ocean; and on account of this continuity, we can convey our thoughts directly to one another.

You see what is happening all around us. The world is one of influence. Part of our energy is used up in the preservation of our own bodies; beyond that, every particle of our energy is day and night being used in influencing others. Our bodies, our virtues, our intellect, and our spirituality—all these are continuously influencing others; and so, conversely, we are being influenced by them. This is going on all around us. Now, to take a concrete example: A man comes. You know he is very learned, his language is beautiful, and he speaks to you by the hour—but he does not make any impression. Another man comes, and he speaks a few words, not well arranged, ungrammatical perhaps; all the same, he makes an immense impression. Many of you have seen that. So it is evident that words alone cannot always produce an impression. Words, even thoughts, contribute only one-third of the influence in making an impression; the man, two-thirds. What you call the personal magnetism of the man—that is what goes out and impresses you.

Each family has a head; some heads of families are successful, others are not. Why? We accuse others for our failures. The moment I am unsuccessful, I say that So-and-so is the cause of the failure. In failures, one does not like to confess one's own faults and weaknesses. Each person tries to hold himself faultless and lay the blame upon somebody or something else, or even on bad luck. When the head of a family fails he should ask himself why it is that some persons manage their families so well and he cannot. Then it will be apparent that the difference is owing to the man—his personality.

Coming to great leaders of mankind, we always find that it was the personality of the man that counted. Now, take all the great authors of the past, the great thinkers. Really, how many original thoughts have they thought? Take all the writings that have been left to us by the past leaders of mankind; take each one of their books and appraise them. The real thoughts, new and genuine, that have been thought in this world up to this time amount to only a handful. Read in their books the thoughts they have left to us. The authors do not appear to be giants to us, and yet we know that they were great giants in their day. What made them so? Not simply the thoughts they thought, neither the books they wrote, nor the speeches they made; it was something else that is now gone, and that is their personality. As I have already remarked, the personality of the man is two-thirds, and his intellect, his words, are but one-third. It is the real man, the personality of the man, that influences us.

Our actions are but effects; actions must come when the man is there; the effect is bound to follow the cause. The ideal of all education, all training, should be this man-making. But instead of that, we are always trying to polish up the outside. What use is there in polishing up the outside when there is no inside? The aim of all training should be to make the man grow. The man who influences, who throws his magic, as it were, upon his fellow beings, is a dynamo of power, and when that man is ready, he can do anything and everything he likes; that personality, handling anything, will make it work.

Now, we see that though this is a fact, no physical laws that we know of will explain it. How can we explain it by the laws of chemistry and physics? How much of oxygen, hydrogen, carbon, how many molecules in different positions, and how many cells, and so on, can explain this mysterious personality? And still we see it is a fact; and not only that, it is the real man; and it is that man that lives and moves and works; it is that man that influences, moves his fellow beings, and passes away; and his intellect and books and works are but traces left behind. Think of this. Compare the great teachers of religion with intellectual philosophers. The latter scarcely influenced anybody's inner self, and yet they wrote most marvellous books. The religious teachers, on the other hand, moved countries in their lifetime. The difference was made by personality. In the philosopher it is a faint personality that influences; in the great prophets it is a tremendous one. In the former we touch the intellect; in the latter we touch life. In the one case it is simply a chemical process, putting certain chemical ingredients together which may gradually combine and, under proper circumstances, bring out a flash of light, or may fail. In the other, it is like a torch that goes round quickly lighting others.

The science of Yoga claims that it has discovered the laws which develop this personality, and by proper attention to those laws and methods each one can grow and strengthen his personality. This is one of the great practical things and this is the secret of all education. It has a universal application: in the life of the householder, in the life of the poor, the rich, the man of business, the spiritual man—in everyone's life—it is a great thing, the strengthening of this personality. As we know, there are laws, very fine, which are behind the physical laws. That is to say, there are no such realities as a physical world, a mental world, a spiritual world. Whatever is, is one. Let us say, it is a sort of tapering existence: the thickest part is here; it tapers and becomes finer and finer. The finest is what we call Spirit; the grossest, the body. And just as it is here, in the microcosm, exactly so is it in the macrocosm. This universe of ours is exactly like that: the thickest part is the gross, external world, and it tapers into something finer and finer until it becomes God.

We also know that the greatest power is lodged in the fine, not in the gross. We see a man take up a huge weight: we see his muscles swell, and all over his body we see signs of exertion; and we think the muscles are powerful things. But it is the thin, thread-like wires, the nerves, which bring power to the muscles; the moment one of these threads is cut off from reaching the muscles, they are not able to work at all. These tiny nerves bring the power from something still finer; and that again in its turn brings it from something finer still—thought; and so on. So it is the fine that is really the seat of power. Of course, we can see the movements in the gross; but when the fine movements take place we cannot see them. When a gross thing moves, we catch it, and thus we naturally identify movement with things which are gross. But all the power is really in the fine.

We do not see any movement in the fine, perhaps because the movement is so intense that we cannot perceive it. But if by any science, any investigation, we are helped to get hold of these finer forces which are the cause of the gross manifestation, the gross itself will be under control. There is a little bubble coming from the bottom of a lake: we do not see it coming all the time; we see it only when it bursts on the surface. So we can perceive thoughts only after they develop a great deal or after they become actions.

We constantly complain that we have no control over our actions, over our thoughts. But how can we have it? If we can get control over the fine movements, if we can get hold of thought at the root, before it has become thought, before it has become action, then it will be possible for us to control the whole. Now, if there is a method by which we can analyse, investigate, understand, and finally grapple with those finer powers, the finer causes, then alone is it possible to have control over ourselves. And the man who has control over his own mind assuredly will have control over every other mind. That is why purity and morality have always been the object of religion. A pure, moral man has control of himself. And all minds are the same—different parts of one Mind. He who knows one lump of clay has known all the clay in the universe. He who knows and controls his own mind knows the secret of every mind and has power over every mind.

Now, we can get rid of a good deal of our physical evil if we have control over the fine parts; we can throw off a good many worries if we have control over the fine movements; a good many failures can be averted if we have control over these fine powers. So far is its utility. Yet beyond there is something higher.

Now I shall tell you a theory. I shall not argue about it but simply place before you the conclusion. Each man in his childhood runs through the stages through which his race has come up; only the race took thousands of years to do it, while the child takes a few years. The child is first the old savage man and, like a savage, he crushes a butterfly under his feet. He is like a primitive ancestor of his race. As he grows, he passes through different stages until he reaches the development of his race; only he does it swiftly and quickly. Now, take the whole of humanity as a race, or take the whole of the animal creation —man and the lower animals as one whole. There is an end towards which the whole is moving. Let us call it perfection. Some men and women there are who anticipate the whole progress of mankind. Instead of waiting and being born over and over again for ages until the whole human race has attained to that perfection, they rush through them, as it were, in the few short years of their life. And we know that we can hasten these processes if we be true to ourselves. If a number of men without any culture are left to live upon an island and are given barely enough food, clothing, and shelter, they will in the course of time evolve higher and higher stages of civilization. But we know also that this growth can be hastened by additional means. We help the growth of trees, do we not? Left to nature they would have grown, only they would have taken longer. We help them to grow in a shorter time than they would otherwise have taken. We are doing all the time the same thing—hastening the growth of things by artificial means.

Why cannot we hasten the growth of man? We can do that as a race. Why are teachers sent to other countries? Because by these means we can hasten the growth of races. Now, cannot we hasten the growth of individuals? We can. Can we put a limit to the hastening process? We cannot say how much a man can grow in one life. You have no reason to say that this much a man can do and no more. Circumstances can hasten his growth wonderfully. Can there be any limit then, till he comes to perfection?

So what comes of this principle? A perfect man, that is to say, the type that is to come of his race perhaps millions of years hence—that man can come today. And this is what the yogis say: that all great Incarnations and prophets are such men; that they reached perfection in this one life. We have had such men at all periods of the world's history and at all times. Quite recently there was such a man who lived the life of the whole human race and reached the end in this very life. Even this hastening of the growth must be under laws. Suppose we investigate these laws and understand their secrets and apply them to our own needs; it follows that we grow. We hasten our growth, we hasten our development, and we become perfect even in this life.

This is the higher part of life, and the science of the study of the mind and its powers has this perfection as its real end. Helping others with money and other material things and teaching them how to go on smoothly in their daily life are secondary. The purpose of this science is to bring out the perfect man and not let him wait and wait for ages, just a plaything in the hands of the physical world, like a log of driftwood carried from wave to wave and tossing about in the ocean. This science wants you to be strong, to take the work in your own hands instead of leaving it in the hands of nature, and get beyond this little life. That is the great idea.

Man is growing in knowledge, in power, in happiness. Continuously we are growing as a race. We see that is true, perfectly true. Is it true of individuals? To a certain extent, yes. But yet, again comes the question: Where do you fix the limit? I can see only for a distance of so many feet. But I have seen a man close his eyes and see what is happening in another room. If you say you do not believe it, perhaps in three weeks that man can make you do the same. It can be taught to anybody. Some persons, in five minutes even, can be made to read what is happening in another man's mind. These facts can be demonstrated.

Now, if these things are true, where can we put a limit? If a man can read what is happening in another's mind in the corner of this room, why not in the next room? Why not anywhere? We cannot say why not. We dare not say that it is not possible. We can only say that we do not know how it happens. Physical scientists have no right to say that things like this are not possible; they can only say, "We do not know." Science has to collect facts, generalize upon them, deduce principles, and state the truth—that is all. But if we begin by denying the facts, how can there be a science?

There is no end to the power a man can obtain. This is the peculiarity of the Indian mind: when anything interests it, it gets absorbed in it and other things are neglected. You know how many sciences had their origin in India. Mathematics began there. You are even today counting one, two, three, and so on, to zero, after Sanskrit figures, and you all know that algebra also originated in India, and that gravitation was known to the Indians centuries before Newton was born.

You see the peculiarity. At a certain period of Indian history this one subject of man and his mind absorbed all the interest of the Hindus. And it was so enticing because it seemed the easiest way to achieve their ends. Now, the Hindus became so thoroughly persuaded that the mind could do anything and everything according to law that its powers became the great object of study. There was nothing extraordinary about charms, magic, and other powers. They were regularly taught, just like the physical sciences they had taught before that. Such a conviction about these things came upon the race that the physical sciences nearly died out. This one thing claimed their attention. Different sects of yogis began to make all sorts of experiments. Some made experiments with light, trying to find out how lights of different colours produced changes in the body. They wore clothes of a certain colour, ate foods of a certain colour, and used things of a certain colour. All sorts of experiments were made in this way. Others made experiments with sound, by stopping and unstopping their ears. And still others experimented with the sense of smell and so on. The whole idea was to reach the source, to reach the fine aspect of the thing. And some of them really attained most marvellous results.

Many of them tried to float in the air or pass through it. I shall tell you a story which I heard from a great scholar in the West. It was told him by a Governor of Ceylon, who saw the performance. A girl was brought forward and seated cross-legged upon a stool made of sticks crossed. After she had been seated for a time, the showman began to take out these cross-bars one after another; and when all were taken out, the girl was left floating in the air. The Governor thought there was some trick; so he drew his sword and violently passed it under the girl. Nothing was there. Now, what was this? It was not magic or something supernatural. That is the peculiarity. No one in India will tell you that things like this do not exist. To the Hindus it is a matter of course. You know what the Hindus would often say when they had to fight their enemies: "Oh, one of our yogis will come and drive them all out!" Perhaps it is going to the extreme. But be that as it may, what power is there in the hand or the sword? The power is all in the Spirit.

If this is true, it is temptation enough for the mind to exert its highest. But just as it is very difficult to make any great achievement in other sciences, so also in this—nay, much more. Yet most people think that these powers can be easily gained. How many are the years you take to make a fortune? Think of that. First, how many years do you take to learn electrical science or engineering? And then you have to work all the rest of your life.

Again, most of the other sciences deal with things that do not move, that are fixed. You can analyse a chair; the chair does not fly from you. But this science deals with the mind, which moves all the time; the moment you want to study it, it slips away. Now the mind is in one mood; the next moment, perhaps, it is different—changing, changing all the time. In the midst of all this change it has to be studied, understood, grasped, and controlled. How much more difficult then is this science! It requires rigorous training. People ask me why I do not give them practical lessons. Why, it is no joke. I stand upon this platform talking to you, and you go home and find no benefit; nor do I. Then you say, "It is all bosh." It is, because you wanted to make bosh of it. I know very little of this science; but the little that I gained I worked for for thirty years of my life, and for six years I have been

telling people the little that I know. It took me thirty
years to learn it—thirty years of hard struggle. Some
times I worked at it twenty hours during the twenty-
four; sometimes I slept only one hour in the night;
sometimes I worked whole nights. Sometimes I lived in
places where there was hardly a sound, hardly a
breath; sometimes I had to live in caves. Think of that.
And yet I know little or nothing; I have barely
touched the hem of the garment of this science. But I
can understand that it is true and vast and wonderful.

Now, if there is anyone among you who really
wants to study this science, he will have to start with
that sort of determination, the same as, nay, even
more than, that which he puts into any business of
life. And what an amount of attention does business
require, and what a rigorous taskmaster it is! Even if
the father, the mother, the wife, or the child dies, the
business cannot stop. Even if the heart is breaking, we
still have to go to our place of business, when every
hour of work is a pang. That is business; and we
think that it is just, that it is right.

This science calls for more application than any
business can ever require. Many men can succeed in
business, very few in this, because so much depends
upon the particular constitution of the person studying
it. As in business all may not make a fortune, but
everyone can make something, so in the study of this
science each one can get a glimpse which will con-
vince him of its truth and of the fact that there have
been men who have realized it fully.

This is an outline of this science. It stands upon its
own feet and in its own light and challenges compari-

son with any other science. There have been charlatans, there have been magicians, there have been
cheats, and more here than in any other field. Why?
For the simple reason that the more profitable the
business, the greater the number of charlatans and
cheats. But that is no reason why the business should
not be good. And one thing more: It may be a good
intellectual gymnastic to listen to all the arguments
and an intellectual satisfaction to hear of wonderful
things. But if any one of you really wants to learn
something beyond that, merely attending lectures will
not do. This cannot be taught in lectures, for it is
life; and only life can convey life. If there are any
among you who are really determined to learn it, I
shall be very glad to help you.

REINCARNATION[1]

"Both you and I have passed through many births.
You know them not; I know them all."
—Bhagavad Gitā.

O F THE MANY RIDDLES that have perplexed the intellect of man in all climes and times, the most
intricate is himself. Of the myriad mysteries that have
called forth his energies to struggle for their solution,
from the very dawn of history, the most mysterious is
his own nature. It is at once the most insoluble enigma
and the problem of all problems. As the starting-point
and the repository of all we know and feel and do,
there never has been, nor will be, a time when man's
own nature will cease to demand his best and foremost attention.

Though through hunger after that truth which of
all others has the most intimate connexion with his
very existence; though through an all-absorbing desire
for an inward standard by which to measure the outward universe; though through the absolute and inherent necessity of finding a fixed point in a universe
of change, man has sometimes clutched at handfuls of
dust for gold, and even when urged on by a voice
higher than reason or intellect has many times failed

[1] Contributed to the *Metaphysical Magazine*, New York,
March 1895.

to interpret rightly the meaning of the divinity within —still there never has been a time, since the search began, when some race or some individuals did not hold aloft the lamp of truth.

Taking a one-sided, cursory, and prejudiced view of the surroundings and the unessential details, sometimes disgusted also with the vagueness of many schools and sects, and often, alas, driven to the opposite extreme by the violent superstitions of organized priestcraft, men have not been wanting, especially among advanced intellects, in either ancient or modern times, who not only have given up the search in despair, but have declared it fruitless and useless. Philosophers may fret and sneer, and priests ply their trade even at the point of the sword; but truth comes to those alone who worship at her shrine for her sake only, without fear and without shopkeeping.

Light comes to individuals through the conscious efforts of their intellects; it comes slowly, though, to the whole race, through unconscious percolation. The philosophers show the volitional struggles of great minds. History reveals the silent process of permeation through which truth is absorbed by the masses.

Of all the theories that have been held by man about himself, that of a soul entity, separate from the body and immortal, has been the most widespread. And among those that have held the belief in such a soul, the majority of the thoughtful have always believed also in its pre-existence. At present the greater portion of the human race with an organized religion believes in it; and many of the best thinkers in the most favoured lands, though nurtured in religions avowedly hostile to every idea of the pre-existence of the soul, have endorsed it. Hinduism and Buddhism have it for their foundation; the educated classes among the ancient Egyptians believed in it; the ancient Persians arrived at it; some of the Greek philosophers made it the corner-stone of their philosophy; the Pharisees among the Hebrews accepted it; and the Sufis, among the Mohammedans, almost universally acknowledged its truth.

There must be peculiar surroundings which generate and foster certain forms of belief among nations. It required ages for the ancient races to arrive at any idea about something apart from the body which survives after death. It took ages more to come to any rational idea about this something which persists and lives apart from the body. It was only when the idea was reached of an entity whose connexion with the body was only for a time, and only among those nations who arrived at such a conclusion, that the unavoidable question arose: Whither? Whence?

The ancient Hebrews never disturbed their equanimity by questioning themselves about the soul. With them death ended all. Karl Heckel justly says: "Though it is true that in the Old Testament, preceding the exile, the Hebrews distinguish a life principle, different from the body, which is sometimes called 'Nephesh,' or 'Ruakh,' or 'Neshama,' yet all these words correspond rather to the idea of breath, than to that of spirit or soul. Also, in the writings of the Palestinian Jews, after the exile, no mention is ever made of an individual immortal soul, but always only of a life-breath emanating from God, which, after the body is dissolved, is reabsorbed into the divine 'Ruakh.'"

The ancient Egyptians and the Chaldeans had peculiar beliefs of their own about the soul; but their ideas about this soul living after death must not be confused with those of the ancient Hindu, the Persian, the Greek, or any other Āryan race. There was from the earliest times a broad distinction between the Āryans and the non-Sanskrit-speaking mlechchas in the conception of the soul. Externally it was typified by their disposal of the dead—the mlechchas mostly trying their best to preserve the dead bodies either by careful burial or by the more elaborate processes of mummifying, and the Āryans generally burning their dead. Herein lies the key to a great secret: the fact that no mlechcha race, whether Egyptian, Assyrian, or Babylonian, ever attained to the idea of the soul as a separate entity which can live independent of the body, without the help of the Āryans, especially of the Hindus.

Although Herodotus states that the Egyptians were the first to conceive the idea of the immortality of the soul, and states, as a doctrine of the Egyptians, that "the soul after the dissolution of the body enters again and again into a creature that comes to life; then, that the soul wanders through all the animals of the land and the sea and through all the birds, and finally, after three thousand years, returns to a human body," yet modern researches into Egyptology have hitherto found no trace of metempsychosis in the popular Egyptian religion. On the contrary, the most recent researches of Maspero, A. Erman, and other eminent

Egyptologists tend to confirm the supposition that the doctrine of palingenesis was not at home with the Egyptians.

With the ancient Egyptians the soul was only a double, having no individuality of its own and never able to break its connexion with the body. It persisted only so long as the body lasted, and if by chance the corpse was destroyed, the departed soul suffered a second death and annihilation. The soul after death was allowed to roam freely all over the world, but it must always return at night to where the corpse was, feeling always miserable, always hungry and thirsty, always extremely desirous to enjoy life once more, and never being able to fulfil the desire. If any part of its old body was injured, the soul was also invariably injured in its corresponding part, and this idea explains the solicitude of the ancient Egyptians to preserve their dead.

At first the deserts were chosen as the burial-place, because the dryness of the air did not allow the body to perish soon, thus granting to the departed soul a long lease of existence. In the course of time one of the gods discovered the process of making mummies, through which the devout hoped to preserve the dead bodies of their ancestors for an almost infinite length of time, thus securing immortality to the departed ghost, however miserable it might be.

The perpetual regret for the world, in which the soul could take no further interest, never ceased to torture the deceased. "O my brother," exclaims the departed, "withhold not thyself from drinking and eating, from drunkenness, from love, from all enjoyment, from following thy desire by night and by day; put not sorrow within thy heart; for what are the years of man upon earth? The west is a land of sleep and of heavy shadows, a place wherein the inhabitants, when once installed, slumber on in their mummy forms, never more waking to see their brethren, never more to recognize their fathers and mothers, with hearts forgetful of their wives and children. The living water which earth giveth to all who dwell upon it is for me stagnant and dead; that water floweth to all who are on earth, while for me it is but liquid putrefaction, this water that is mine. Since I came into this funeral valley I know not where nor what I am. Give me to drink of running water, . . . let me be placed by the edge of the water with my face to the north, that the breeze may caress me and my heart be refreshed from its sorrow."[2]

Among the Chaldeans also, although they did not speculate so much as the Egyptians as to the condition of the soul after death, the soul was still a double and was bound to its sepulchre. They also could not conceive of a state without this physical body, and expected a resurrection of the corpse again to life; and though the goddess Ishtar, after great perils and adventures, procured the resurrection of her shepherd husband Dumuzi, the son of Ea and Damkina, "the most pious votaries pleaded in vain from temple to temple for the resurrection of their dead friends."

Thus we find that the ancient Egyptians and

[2] This text has been translated into German by Brugsch, *Die Egyptische Gräberwelt*, pp. 39-40, and into French by Maspero, *Études Égyptiennes*, Vol. I, pp. 181-190.

Chaldeans never could entirely dissociate the idea of the soul from the corpse of the departed or from the sepulchre. The state of earthly existence was best after all, and the departed were always longing to have a chance once more to renew it; and the living were fervently hoping to help them in prolonging the existence of the miserable double and striving the best they could to help them.

This is not the soil out of which any higher knowledge of the soul can spring. In the first place the whole idea is grossly materialistic, and even then it is one of terror and agony. Frightened by the almost innumerable powers of evil, and making hopeless, agonized efforts to avoid them, the souls of the living, like their ideas of the souls of the departed—wander all over the world though they might—could never get beyond the sepulchre and the crumbling corpse.

We must turn now for the source of the higher ideas of the soul to another race, whose God was an all-merciful, all-pervading Being manifesting Himself through various bright, benign, and helpful devas; the first of all the human race who addressed their God as Father: "Oh, take me by the hands even as a father takes his dear son"; with whom life was a hope and not a despair; whose religion was not the intermittent groans escaping from the lips of an agonized man during the intervals of a life of mad excitement, but whose ideas come to us redolent with the aroma of the field and forest; whose songs of praise—spontaneous, free, joyful, like the songs which burst forth from the throats of the birds when they hail this beautiful world illuminated by the first rays of the lord of the day—

come down to us even now, through the vista of eighty centuries, as fresh calls from heaven. We turn to the ancient Āryans.

"Place me in that deathless, undecaying world where is the light of heaven and everlasting lustre shines"; "Make me immortal in that realm where dwells King Vivasvān's son, where is the secret shrine of heaven"; "Make me immortal in that realm where they move even as they list"; "In the third sphere of the inmost heaven, where the worlds are full of light, make me immortal in that realm of bliss"—these are the prayers of the Āryans in their oldest record, the Rig-Veda Samhitā.

We find at once a whole world of difference between the mlechcha and the Āryan ideals. To the one, this body and this world were all that were real and all that were desirable. A little life-fluid which flew off from the body at death, to feel torture and agony at the loss of the enjoyments of the senses, could, they fondly hoped, be brought back if the body was carefully preserved; and thus the corpse became more of an object of care than the living man. The other found out that that which left the body was the real man, and when separated from the body it enjoyed a state of bliss higher than it ever enjoyed when in the body; and they hastened to annihilate the corrupted corpse by burning it.

Here we find the germ out of which a true idea of the soul could come. Here it was—where the real man was not the body, but the soul; where all ideas of an inseparable connexion between the real man and the body were utterly absent—that a noble idea of the freedom of the soul could arise. And it was when the Āryans penetrated even beyond the shining cloth of the body with which the departed soul was enveloped, and found its real nature, a formless, individual principle, that the question inevitably arose: Whence?

It was in India and among the Āryans that the doctrine of the pre-existence, the immortality, and the individuality of the soul first arose. Recent researches in Egypt have failed to show any trace of the doctrines of an independent and individual soul existing before and after the earthly phase of existence. Some of the mysteries were no doubt in possession of this idea, but in those it has been traced to India.

"I am convinced," says Karl Heckel, "that the deeper we enter into the study of the Egyptian religion, the more clearly it is shown that the doctrine of metempsychosis was entirely foreign to the popular Egyptian religion, and that even that which single mysteries possessed of it was not inherent in the Osiris teachings, but derived from Hindu sources."

Later on we find the Alexandrian Jews imbued with the doctrine of an individual soul; and the Pharisees of the time of Jesus, as already stated, not only had faith in an individual soul, but believed in its wanderings through various bodies; and thus it is easy to find how Christ was recognized as the incarnation of an older prophet, and Jesus himself directly asserted that John the Baptist was the prophet Elias come back again. "If ye will receive it, this is Elias, which was for to come." (Matt. 11:14.)

The idea of a soul and of its individuality, among the Hebrews, evidently came through the higher mystical teachings of the Egyptians, who in their turn had derived it from India. And that it should come through Alexandria is significant, since the Buddhist records clearly show Buddhist missionary activity in Alexandria and Asia Minor.

Pythagoras is said to have been the first Greek who taught the doctrine of palingenesis among the Hellenes. As an Āryan race, already burning their dead and believing in the doctrine of an individual soul, it was easy for the Greeks to accept the doctrine of reincarnation, through the Pythagorean teachings. According to Apuleius, Pythagoras had gone to India, where he had been instructed by the brāhmins.

So far we have learnt that wherever the soul was held to be an individual, the real man, and not a vivifying part of the body only, the doctrine of its pre-existence inevitably came, and that those nations that believed in the independent individuality of the soul almost always signified it externally by burning the bodies of the departed; though one of the ancient Āryan races, the Persian, developed at an early period, and without any Semitic influence, a peculiar method of disposing of the bodies of the dead; the very name by which they call their "towers of silence" comes from the Sanskrit root *daha,* to burn.

In short, the races who did not pay much attention to the analysis of their own nature never went beyond the material body as their all in all; and even when driven by higher light to penetrate beyond, they only came to the conclusion that somehow or other, at some distant period of time, this body will become incorruptible. On the other hand, that race which spent the best part of its energies in the inquiry into the nature of man as a thinking being—the Indo-Āryan— soon found out that beyond this body, beyond even the shining body which their forefathers longed for, is the real man, the principle, the individual who clothes himself with this body and then throws it off when worn out.

Was such a principle created? If creation means something coming out of nothing, the answer is a decisive no. This soul is without birth and without death. It is not a compound or combination, but an independent individual, and as such it cannot be created or destroyed; it is only travelling through various states.

Naturally, the question arises: Where was it all this time? The Hindu philosophers say that in the physical sense it was passing through different bodies, or, really and metaphysically speaking, passing through different mental planes.

Are there any proofs, apart from the teachings of the Vedas, upon which the doctrine of reincarnation has been founded by the Hindu philosophers? There are; and we hope to show later on that there are grounds as valid for it as for any universally accepted doctrine. But first we shall see what some of the greatest of modern European thinkers have thought about reincarnation.

Schopenhauer, in his book *Die Welt als Wille und Vorstellung*, speaking about palingenesis, says:

"What sleep is for the individual, death is for the 'will.' It would not endure to continue the same actions and sufferings throughout an eternity without true gain, if memory and individuality remained to it. It flings them off, and this is Lethe, and through this sleep of death it reappears fitted out with another intellect as a new being; a new day tempts to new shores. These constant new births, then, constitute the succession of the life-dreams of a will which in itself is indestructible, until, instructed and improved by so much and such various successive knowledge in a constantly new form, it abolishes and abrogates itself. . . . It must not be neglected that even empirical grounds support a palingenesis of this kind. As a matter of fact, there does exist a connexion between the birth of the newly appearing beings and the death of those that are worn out. It shows itself in the great fruitfulness of the human race which appears as a consequence of devastating diseases. When in the fourteenth century the Black Death had for the most part depopulated the Old World, a quite abnormal fruitfulness appeared among the human race, and twin-births were very frequent. The circumstance was also remarkable that none of the children born at this time obtained their full number of teeth; thus nature, exerting itself to the utmost, was niggardly in details. This is related by F. Schnurrer in his *Chronik der Seuchen*, 1825. Casper also, in his *Über die Wahrscheinliche Lebensdauer des Menschen*, 1835, confirms the principle that the number of births in a given population has the most decided influence upon the length of life and mortality in it, as this always keeps pace with mortality; so that always and everywhere the deaths and the births increase and decrease in like proportion, which he places beyond doubt by an accumulation of evidence collected from many lands and their various provinces. And yet it is impossible that there can be a physical, causal connexion between my early death and the fruitfulness of a marriage with which I have nothing to do, or conversely. Thus here the metaphysical appears undeniable, and in a stupendous manner, as the immediate ground of explanation of the physical. Every newborn being comes fresh and blithe into the new existence, and enjoys it as a free gift; but there is and can be nothing freely given. Its fresh existence is paid for by the old age and death of a worn-out existence which has perished, but which contained the indestructible seed out of which the new existence has arisen; they are one being."

The great English philosopher Hume, nihilistic though he was, says in the sceptical essay on immortality: "The metempsychosis is therefore the only system of this kind that philosophy can listen to." The philosopher Lessing, with a deep poetical insight, asks: "Is this hypothesis so laughable merely because it is the oldest? because the human understanding, before the sophistries of the schools had dissipated and debilitated it, lighted upon it at once? . . . Why should not I come back as often as I am capable of acquiring fresh knowledge, fresh experience? Do I bring away so much from one life that there is nothing to repay the trouble of coming back?"

The arguments for and against the doctrine of a pre-existing soul reincarnating through many lives have been many, and some of the greatest thinkers of all ages have taken up the gauntlet to defend it; and so far as we can see, if there is an individual soul, that it existed before seems inevitable. If the soul is not an individual, but a combination of skandhas, or notions, as the Mādhyamikas among the Buddhists insist, still they find pre-existence absolutely necessary to explain their position.

The argument showing the impossibility of an infinite existence's beginning in time is unanswerable, though attempts have been made to ward it off by appealing to the power of God to do anything, however contrary to reason it may be. We are sorry to find this most fallacious argument proceeding from some of the most thoughtful persons.

In the first place, God being the universal and common cause of all phenomena, the question was to find the natural causes of certain phenomena in the human soul, and the *deus ex machina* theory is therefore quite irrelevant. It amounts to nothing more than confession of ignorance. We can give that answer to every question asked in every branch of human knowledge, and stop all inquiry, and therefore knowledge, altogether.

Secondly, this constant appeal to the omnipotence of God is only a word-puzzle. The cause, as cause, is and can only be known to us as sufficient for the effect, and nothing more. As such we have no more idea of an infinite effect than of an omnipotent cause. Moreover, all our ideas of God are limited; even the idea of cause limits our idea of God. Thirdly, even taking the position for granted, we are not bound to allow any such absurd theories as "something coming out of nothing" or "infinity beginning in time" so long as we can give a better explanation.

A so-called strong argument is made against the idea of pre-existence by asserting that the majority of mankind are not conscious of it. To prove the validity of this argument, the person who offers it must prove that the whole of the soul of man is bound up in the faculty of memory. If memory be the test of existence, then all that part of our lives which is not now in it must be non-existent, and every person who in a state of coma, or otherwise, loses his memory must be non-existent also.

The premises from which the inference is drawn of a previous existence, and that, too, on the plane of conscious action, as adduced by the Hindu philosophers, are chiefly these:

First, how else do you explain this world of inequalities? Here is one child born in the providence of a just and merciful God, with every circumstance conducing to his becoming a good and useful member of the human race, and perhaps at the same instant and in the same city another child is born, under circumstances every one of which is against his becoming good. We see children born to suffer, perhaps all their lives, and that owing to no fault of theirs. Why should it be so? What is the cause? Of whose ignorance is it the result? If not the child's, why should it suffer? For its parents' actions?

It is much better to confess ignorance than try to evade the question by the allurements of future enjoyments in proportion to the evil here, or by posing "mysteries." Not only undeserved suffering forced upon us by any agent is immoral—not to say unjust—but even the future-making-up theory has no legs to stand upon. How many of the miserably born struggle towards a higher life, and how many more succumb to the circumstances they are placed under? Should those who grow worse and more wicked by being forced to be born under evil circumstances be rewarded for the wickedness of their lives in the future? In that case, the more wicked the man is here, the better will be his deserts hereafter.

There is no other way to vindicate the glory and the liberty of the human soul and to reconcile the inequalities and the horrors of this world than to place the whole burden upon the legitimate cause: our own independent actions, or karma. Not only so, but every theory of the creation of the soul from nothing inevitably leads to fatalism and preordination, and instead of a merciful Father, places before us a hideous, cruel, and ever angry God to worship. And so far as the power of religion for good or evil is concerned, this theory of a created soul, leading to its corollaries of fatalism and predestination, is responsible for the horrible idea prevailing among Christians and Mohammedans that the heathen are the lawful victims of their swords, and for all the horrors that have followed and are following it still.

But an argument which the philosophers of the Nyāya school have always advanced in favour of reincarnation, and which to us seems conclusive, is this: Our experiences cannot be annihilated. Our actions (karma), though apparently disappearing, remain still unperceived (adrishtam), and reappear again in their effect as tendencies (pravrittis). Even little babies come with certain tendencies: fear of death, for example.

Now, if a tendency is the result of repeated actions, the tendencies with which we are born must be explained on that ground too. Evidently we could not have got them in this life; therefore we have to seek for their genesis in the past. Now, it is also evident that some of our tendencies are the effects of the self-conscious efforts peculiar to man; and if it is true that we are born with such tendencies, it rigorously follows that their causes were conscious efforts in the past—that is, we must have been on the same mental plane which we call the human plane before this present life.

So far as explaining the tendencies of the present life by past conscious efforts goes, the reincarnationists of India and the latest school of evolutionists are at one; the only difference is that the Hindus, being spiritual, explain them by the conscious efforts of individual souls, and the materialistic school of evolutionists, by hereditary physical transmission. The schools which hold to the theory of creation out of nothing are entirely out of court.

The issue has to be fought out between the reincarnationists, who hold that all experiences are stored up as tendencies in the subject of those experiences, the individual soul, and are transmitted by reincarnation of that unbroken individuality, and the materialists, who hold that the brain is the subject of all actions and accept the theory of transmission through cells.

Thus the doctrine of reincarnation assumes an infinite importance to our mind; for the fight between reincarnation and mere cellular transmission is, in reality, the fight between spirituality and materialism. If cellular transmission is the all-sufficient explanation, materialism is inevitable and there is no necessity for the theory of a soul. If it is not a sufficient explanation, the theory of an individual soul bringing into this life the experiences of the past is as absolutely true. There is no escape from the alternative, reincarnation or materialism. Which shall we accept?

DISCIPLESHIP

(Delivered in San Francisco, March 29, 1900)

MY SUBJECT is "Discipleship." I do not know how you will take what I have to say. It will be rather difficult for you to accept it: the idea of teacher and disciple in this country differs so much from that in ours. An old proverb of India comes to my mind: "There are hundreds of thousands of teachers, but it is hard to find one disciple." It seems to be true. The one important thing in the attainment of spirituality is the attitude of the pupil. When the right attitude is there, illumination comes easily.

What does the disciple need in order to receive the truth? The great sages say that to attain truth takes but the twinkling of an eye: it is just a question of knowing. The dream breaks—how long does it take? In a second the dream is gone. When the illusion vanishes, how long does it take? Just the twinkling of an eye. When I know the truth, nothing happens except that the falsehood vanishes away. I took the rope for a snake, and now I see it is a rope. It is only a question of half a second and the whole thing is done. Thou art That; Thou art Reality—how long does it take to know this? If we are God and always have been so, not to know this is most astonishing. To know this is the only natural thing. It should not take ages to find out what we have always been and what we now are.

Yet it seems difficult to realize this self-evident truth. Ages and ages pass before we begin to catch a faint glimpse of it. God is life; God is truth—we write about this; we feel in our inmost heart that this is so, that everything else but God is nothing—here today, gone tomorrow. And yet most of us remain the same all through life. We cling to untruth and we turn our backs upon truth. We do not want to attain truth. We do not want anyone to break our dream. You see, teachers are not wanted. Who wants to learn? But if anyone wants to realize the truth and overcome illusion, if he wants to receive the truth from a teacher, he must be a true disciple.

It is not easy to be a disciple: great preparations are necessary; many conditions have to be fulfilled. Four principal conditions are laid down by the Vedāntists.

The first condition is that the student who wants to know the truth must give up all desires for gain in this world or in the life to come.

The truth is not what we see. We do not see the truth as long as any desire creeps into the mind. God is true and the world is not true. So long as there is in the heart the least desire for the world, truth will not come. Let the world fall to ruin before my eyes—I do not care. So with the next life: I do not care to go to heaven. What is heaven? Only the continuation of this earth. We would be better off and the little foolish dreams we are dreaming would break sooner if there were no heaven, no continuation of this silly life on earth. By going to heaven we only prolong the miserable illusions.

What do you gain in heaven? You become gods, drink nectar, and get rheumatism! There is less misery there than on earth, but also less truth. The very rich can understand truth much less than the poorer people. "It is easier for a camel to go through the eye of a needle than for a rich man to enter into the kingdom of God." The rich man has no time to think of anything beyond his wealth and power, his comforts and indulgences. The rich rarely become religious. Why? Because they think if they become religious they will have no more fun in life. In the same way, there is very little chance to become spiritual in heaven. There is too much comfort and enjoyment there; the dwellers in heaven are disinclined to give up their fun.

They say there will be no more weeping in heaven. I do not trust the man who never weeps; he has a big block of granite where his heart should be. It is evident that the heavenly people have not much sympathy. There are vast masses of them over there, and we are miserable creatures suffering in this horrible place. They could pull us all out of it, but they do not. They do not weep. There is no sorrow or misery there; therefore they do not care for anyone's misery. They drink their nectar; dances go on—beautiful wives and all that.

Going beyond these things, the disciple should say: "I do not care for anything in this life nor for all the heavens that have ever existed. I do not care to go to any of them. I do not want the sense life in any form

—this identification of myself with the body. As I feel now, I am this body—this mass of flesh; this is what I feel I am. But I refuse to accept that as the final truth."

The world and the heavens, all these are bound up with the senses. You do not care for the world if you do not have any senses. Heaven also is in the world. Earth, heaven, and all that is between have but one name: the world. Therefore the disciple, knowing the past and the present and thinking of the future, knowing what prosperity means, what happiness means, gives up all these and seeks to know truth and truth alone. This is the first condition.

The second condition is that the disciple must be able to control the internal and the external senses and must be established in several other spiritual virtues.

The external senses are the visible organs situated in different parts of the body; the internal senses are intangible. We have the external eyes, ears, nose, and so on, and we have the corresponding internal senses. We are continually at the beck and call of both these groups of senses. Corresponding to the senses are sense-objects. If any sense-objects are near by, the senses compel us to perceive them; we have no choice or independence. There is the big nose. A little fragrance is there: I have to smell it. If there were a bad odour, I would say to myself, "Do not smell it." But the nose says, "Smell," and I smell it. Just think what we have become! We have bound ourselves. I have eyes. Anything going on, good or bad, I must see. It is the same with hearing. If anyone speaks unpleasantly to me, I must hear it. My sense of hearing compels me to do so, and how miserable I feel! Curse or praise man has got to hear. I have seen many deaf people who do not usually hear; but anything about themselves they always hear!

All these senses, external and internal, must be under the disciple's control. By hard practice he has to arrive at the stage where he can assert himself against the senses, against the commands of his mind. He must be able to say to his mind, "You are mine; I order you, do not see or hear anything," and the mind will not see or hear anything—no form or sound will react on the mind. In that state the mind has become free of the domination of the senses, has become separated from them. No longer is it attached to the senses and the body; external things cannot order the mind now; the mind refuses to attach itself to them. There is a beautiful fragrance. The disciple says to the mind, "Do not smell," and the mind does not perceive the fragrance. When you have arrived at that point, you are just beginning to be a disciple. That is why when everybody says, "I know the truth," I say, "If you know the truth, you must have self-control, and if you have control of yourself, show it by controlling the organs."

Next, the mind must be made to quiet down. It is rushing about. Just as I sit down to meditate, all the vilest ideas in the world come up. The whole thing is nauseating. Why should the mind think thoughts I do not want it to think? I am as it were a slave to the mind. No spiritual knowledge is possible so long as the mind is restless and out of control. The disciple has to learn to control the mind. Yes, it is the function of the mind to think. But it must not think if the disciple does not want it to; it must stop thinking when he commands it to. To qualify as a disciple, this state of the mind is very necessary.

Also, the disciple must have great power of endurance. You will find the mind behaving well when everything goes right with you and life seems comfortable. But if something goes wrong, your mind loses its balance. That is not good. Bear all evil and misery without the slightest murmur, without one thought of unhappiness, resistance, remedy, or retaliation. That is true endurance, and that you must acquire.

Good and evil there always are in the world. Many forget there is any evil—at least they try to forget—and when evil comes upon them they are overwhelmed by it and feel bitter. There are others who deny that there is any evil at all and consider everything good. That also is a weakness; that also proceeds from a fear of evil. If something is evil-smelling, why sprinkle it with rose-water and call it fragrant? Yes, there are good and evil in the world. God has put evil in the world. But you do not have to whitewash it. Why there is evil is none of your business. Have faith and keep quiet.

When my Master, Śri Ramakrishna, fell ill, a brāhmin suggested to him that he apply his tremendous mental power to cure himself; he said that if my Master would only concentrate his mind on the diseased part of the body, it would heal. Sri Ramakrishna answered, "What! Bring down the mind that I've given to God to this little body!" He refused to think of body and illness. His mind was continually conscious of God; it was dedicated to Him utterly. He would not use it for any other purpose.

This craving for health, wealth, long life, and the like—the so-called good—is nothing but delusion. To devote the mind to them in order to secure them only strengthens the delusion. We have these dreams and illusions in life, and we want to have more of them in the life to come, in heaven. More and more illusion!

Resist not evil. Face it. You are higher than evil. There is this misery in the world; it has to be suffered by someone. You cannot act without creating evil for somebody. And when you seek worldly good you only avoid an evil which must be suffered by somebody else. Everyone is trying to put it on someone else's shoulders. The disciple says: "Let the miseries of the world come to me; I shall endure them all. Let others go free."

Remember the man on the Cross? He could have brought legions of angels to win him the victory. But he did not resist; he blessed those who crucified him. He endured every humiliation and suffering. He took the burden of all upon himself: "Come unto me, all ye that labour and are heavy laden, and I will give you rest." Such is true endurance. How very high he was above this life, so high that we cannot understand it, we slaves! No sooner does a man slap me in the face than my hand hits back: bang, it goes! How can I understand the greatness and blessedness of the Crucified One? How can I see his glory?

But I will not drag the ideal down. I feel I am the body, resisting evil. If I get a headache, I go all over the world to have it cured. I drink two thousand bottles of medicine. How can I understand these marvellous minds? I can see the ideal—but how much of that ideal? None of this consciousness of the body, of the little self, of its pleasures and pains, its hurts and comforts—none of these can touch that ideal. By thinking only of the Spirit and keeping the mind out of matter all the time, I can catch a glimpse of that ideal. Material thought and forms of the sense-world have no place in that ideal. Put them away and fix the mind upon the Spirit. Forget your life and death, your pains and pleasures, your name and fame, and realize that you are neither body nor mind, but pure Spirit.

When I say "I," I mean this Spirit. Close your eyes and see what picture appears when you think of your "I." Is it the picture of your body that comes, or of your mental nature? If so, you have not realized your true "I" yet. The time will come, however, when as soon as you say "I" you will see the universe, the Infinite Being. Then you will have realized your true Self and found that you are the Infinite. That is the truth. You are the Spirit; you are not matter. There is such a thing as illusion; on account of it one thing is taken for another—matter is taken for Spirit, the body for the Soul. That is the tremendous illusion. It has to go.

The next qualification is that the disciple must have faith in the guru, the teacher. In the West the teacher simply gives intellectual knowledge; that is all. In India the relationship with the teacher is the greatest in life. My guru is my nearest and dearest relative in life; next, my mother, then my father. My first reverence is to my guru. If my father says, "Do this," and my guru says, "Do not do this," I do not do it. The guru frees my soul. The father and mother give me this body, but the guru gives me rebirth in the Spirit.

We have certain peculiar beliefs. One of these is that there are some souls, a few exceptional ones, who are already free and who are born here for the good of the world, to help the world. They are free already. They do not care for their own salvation; they want to help others. They do not require to be taught anything. From their childhood they know everything; they may speak the highest truth even when they are mere babies.

Upon these free souls depends the spiritual growth of mankind. They are like the first lamps from which other lamps are lighted. True, the light is in everyone; but in most men it is hidden. The great souls are shining lamps from their very birth. Those who come in contact with them get, as it were, their own lamps lighted. By this the first lamps do not lose anything, yet they communicate their light to other lamps. A million lamps are lighted, but the first lamps go on shining with undiminished light. One such first lamp is the guru, and the lamp lighted from it is the disciple. The second in turn becomes a guru, and so on. Those great ones whom you call Incarnations of God are mighty spiritual giants. They come and set in motion a tremendous spiritual current by transmitting their power to their immediate disciples, and through them to generation after, generation of disciples.

A bishop in the Christian Church, by the laying on

of hands, claims to transmit the power which he is supposed to have received from the preceding bishops. The bishop says that Jesus Christ transmitted his power to his immediate disciples, and they to others, and that that is how Christ's power has come to him. We hold that every one of us, not bishops only, ought to have such power. There is no reason why each of you cannot be a vehicle of the mighty current of spirituality.

But first you must find a teacher, a true teacher, and you must remember that he is not just a man. You may get a teacher in the body, but the real teacher is not in the body. He is not the physical man; he is not as he appears to your eyes. It may be that the teacher will come to you as a human being, and you will receive the power from him. Sometimes he will come in a dream and transmit the spiritual ideal to you. The power of the teacher may come to us in many ways. But for us ordinary mortals a human teacher must come, and our preparation must go on till he comes.

We attend lectures and read books, argue and reason about God and soul, religion and salvation. This is not spirituality, because spirituality does not exist in books or in theories or in philosophies. It is not in learning or reasoning, but in actual inner growth. Even parrots can learn things by heart and repeat them. If you become learned, what of it? Asses can carry whole libraries. So when real light comes there will be no more of this learning from books— no book-learning. The man who cannot write even his own name can be perfectly religious, and the man with all the libraries of the world in his head may fail to

be so. Learning is not a condition of spiritual growth;
scholarship is not a condition. The touch of the guru,
the transmittal of spiritual energy, will quicken your
heart. Then will begin the growth. That is the real
baptism by fire. No more stopping; you go on and on.

Some years ago one of your Christian teachers, a
friend of mine, said, "You believe in Christ?" "Yes," I
answered, "but perhaps with a little more reverence."
"Then why don't you be baptised?" How could I be
baptised? By whom? Where is the man who can give
true baptism? What is baptism? Is it sprinkling some
water over you or dipping you in water, while mutter-
ing formulas?

Baptism is the direct introduction into the life of
the Spirit. If you receive the real baptism, you know
you are not the body but the Spirit. Give me that
baptism if you can, or else you are not a Christian
teacher. Even after the so-called baptism which you
received, you have remained the same. What is the
sense of merely saying you have been baptised in the
name of Christ? Mere talk—only disturbing the world
with your foolishness! "Ever steeped in the darkness of
ignorance, yet considering themselves wise and learned,
fools go round and round, staggering to and fro like
the blind led by the blind." Therefore do not say you
are Christians, do not brag about baptism and things
of that sort.

Of course there is true baptism. There was baptism
in the beginning when Christ came to the earth and
taught. The illumined souls, the great ones that come
to earth from time to time, have the power to reveal
the supernal vision to us. This is true baptism. You

see, before the forms and ceremonies of any religion come into being, there exists in it the germ of universal truth. In the course of time this truth becomes forgotten; it becomes strangled, as it were, by forms and ceremonies. The forms alone remain—we find only the casket with the spirit gone. You have the form of baptism, but few can evoke the living spirit of baptism. The form will not suffice. If we want to gain the living knowledge of the living truth, we have to be truly initiated into it. That is the ideal.

The guru must teach me and lead me into light, make me a link in that chain of which he himself is a link. The man in the street cannot claim to be a guru. The guru must be a man who has known, has actually realized the Divine Truth, has perceived himself as the Spirit. A mere talker cannot be a guru. A talkative fool like me can talk much, but cannot be a guru. A true guru will tell the disciple, "Go and sin no more," and no more can he sin—no more has the person the power to sin.

I have seen such men in this life. I have read the Bible and all such books; they are wonderful. But the living power you cannot find in books. The power that can transform life in a moment can be found only in living illumined souls, those shining lights who appear among us from time to time. They alone are fit to be gurus. You and I are only hollow talkers, not teachers. We are disturbing the world by talking, making bad vibrations. Let us hope and pray and struggle on, and the day will come when we shall arrive at the truth, and we shall not have to speak.

"The teacher was a boy of sixteen; he taught a man

of eighty. Silence was the method of the teacher, and the doubts of the disciple vanished for ever." That is the guru. Just think: if you find such a man, what faith and love you ought to have for that person! Why, he is God Himself, nothing less than that. That is why Christ's disciples worshipped him as God. The disciple must worship the guru as God Himself. All a man can know is the living God, God as embodied in man, until he himself has realized God. How else would he know God?

Here is a man in America, born nineteen hundred years after Christ, who does not even belong to the same race as Christ, the Jewish race. He has not seen Jesus or his family. He says: "Jesus was God. If you do not believe it, you will go to hell." We can understand how the disciples believed it—that Christ was God; he was their guru and they must have believed he was God. But what has this American got to do with the man born nineteen hundred years ago? This young man tells me that I do not believe in Jesus and therefore I shall have to go to hell. What does he know of Jesus? He is fit for a lunatic asylum. This kind of belief won't do. He will have to find his guru.

Jesus may be born again, may come to you. Then, if you worship him as God, you are all right. We must all wait till the guru comes, and the guru must be worshipped as God. He is God; he is nothing less than that. As you look at him, the guru gradually melts away—and what is left? The picture of the guru gives place to God Himself. The guru is the bright mask which God wears in order to come to us. As we look steadily on him, gradually the mask falls off and God is revealed.

"I bow to the guru, who is the embodiment of the Bliss Divine, the personification of the highest Knowledge, and the giver of the greatest beatitude; who is pure, perfect, one and without a second, eternal, beyond pleasure and pain, beyond all thought and all qualification, transcendental." Such is in reality the guru. No wonder the disciple looks upon him as God Himself and trusts him, reveres him, obeys him, follows him unquestioningly. This is the relation between the guru and the disciple.

The next condition the disciple must fulfil is to conceive an extreme desire to be free.

We are like moths, plunging into the flaming fire of the senses, though fully knowing that it will burn us. Sense enjoyment only enhances our desire. Desire is never satiated by enjoyment; enjoyment only increases desire, as butter fed into fire increases the fire. Desire is increased by desire. Knowing all this, people still plunge into it all the time. Life after life they have been going after the objects of desire, suffering extremely in consequence; yet they cannot give up desire. Even religion, which should rescue them from this terrible bondage to desire, they have made a means of satisfying desire. Rarely do they ask God to free them from bondage to the body and senses, from slavery to desire. Instead they pray to Him for health and prosperity, for long life: "O God, cure my headache, give me some money or something!" The circle of vision has become so narrow, so degraded, so beastly! None is desiring anything beyond this body. Oh, the terrible degradation, the terrible misery of it! Of what little consequence are the flesh, the five senses, the stomach!

What is the world but a combination of stomach and sex? Look at the millions of men and women— that is what they are living for. Take these away from them and they will find their life empty, meaningless, and intolerable. Such are we—and such is our mind. It is continually hankering for ways and means to satisfy the hunger of the stomach and sex. All the time this is going on. There is also endless suffering. These desires of the body bring only momentary satisfaction and endless suffering. It is like drinking a cup of which the surface layer is nectar, while underneath all is poison. But we still hanker for all these things.

What can be done? Renunciation of the senses and of desire is the only way out of this misery. If you want to be spiritual, you must renounce. This is the real test. Give up the world—this nonsense of the senses. There is only one real desire: to know what is true, to be spiritual. No more of materialism, no more of this egoism. I must become spiritual. Strong, intense, must be the desire. If a man's hands and feet were so tied that he could not move, and then if a burning piece of charcoal were placed on his body, he would struggle with all his power to throw it off. When I shall have that sort of extreme desire, that restless struggle to throw off this burning world, then the time will have come for me to glimpse the Divine Truth.

Look at me. If I lose my little pocketbook with two or three dollars in it, I go twenty times into the house to find that pocketbook. The anxiety, the worry, and the struggle! If one of you curses me, I remember it twenty years; I cannot forgive and forget it. For the little things of the senses I can struggle like that.

Who is there that struggles for God that way? "Children forget everything in their play. The young are mad after the enjoyment of the senses; they do not care for anything else. The old are brooding over their past misdeeds." They are thinking of their past enjoyments—old men who cannot have any enjoyment. Chewing the cud—that is the best they can do. None crave for the Lord in the same intense spirit in which they crave for the things of the senses.

They all say that God is the Truth, the only thing that really exists—that Spirit alone is, not matter. Yet the things they seek of God are rarely Spirit. They ask always for material things. In their prayers Spirit is not separated from matter. Degradation—that is what religion has turned out to be. The whole thing is becoming a sham; and the years are rolling on and nothing spiritual is being attained. But man should hunger for one thing alone, the Spirit, because Spirit alone is real. That is the ideal. If you cannot attain it now, say, "I cannot do it; that is the ideal, I know, but I cannot follow it yet." But that is not what you do. You degrade religion to your low level and seek matter in the name of Spirit. You are all atheists. You do not believe in anything except the senses. "So-and-so said such-and-such a thing—there may be something to it. Let us try it out and have the fun. Possibly some benefit will come; possibly my broken leg will get straight."

Miserable are the diseased people; they are great worshippers of the Lord, for they hope that if they pray to Him He will heal them. Not that that is altogether bad—if such prayers are honest and if they remember that that is not religion. Śri Krishna says in the Gitā: "Four classes of people worship Me: the distressed, the seeker of material things, the inquirer, and the knower of Truth." People who are in distress approach God for relief. If they are ill they worship Him to be healed; if they lose their wealth they pray to Him to get it back. There are other people who ask Him for all kinds of things, because they are full of desires—for name, fame, wealth, position, and so on. They will say: "O Virgin Mary, I will make an offering to you if I get what I want. If you are successful in granting my prayer, I will worship God and give you a part of everything." Men not so material as that, but still with no faith in God, feel inclined to know about Him. They study philosophies, read scriptures, listen to lectures, and so on. They are the inquirers. The last class are those who worship God and know Him. All these four classes of people are good, not bad. All of them worship Him.

But we are trying to be disciples. Our sole concern is to know the highest Truth. Our goal is the loftiest. We have said big words to ourselves—absolute realization and all that. Let us measure up to the words. Let us worship the Spirit in Spirit, standing on Spirit. Let the foundation be Spirit; the middle, Spirit; the culmination, Spirit. There will be no world anywhere. Let it go and whirl into space—who cares? Stand thou upon the Spirit! That is the goal. We know we cannot reach it yet. Never mind. Do not despair, and do not drag the ideal down. The important thing is how much less you think of the body, of yourself, as matter, as dead, dull, insentient matter; how much more you think of yourself as shining, immortal Being. The more you think of yourself as shining, immortal Spirit, the more eager you will be to be absolutely free of matter, body, and senses. This is the intense desire to be free.

The fourth and last condition of discipleship is the discrimination of the Real from the unreal. There is only one thing that is real: God. All the time the mind must be drawn to Him, dedicated to Him. God exists; nothing else exists. Everything else comes and goes. Any desire for the world is illusion, because the world is unreal. More and more the mind must become conscious of God alone, until everything else appears as it really is: unreal.

These are the four conditions which one who wants to be a disciple must fulfil. Without fulfilling them he will not be able to come in contact with a true guru. And even if he is fortunate enough to find one, he will not be quickened by the power that the guru may transmit. There cannot be any compromising of these conditions. With the fulfilment of these conditions—with all these preparations—the lotus of the disciple's heart will open and the bee will come. Then the disciple knows that the real guru was within the body, within himself. He unfolds. He realizes the Spirit. He crosses the ocean of life, goes beyond. He crosses this terrible ocean, and in mercy, without a thought of gain or praise, he in his turn helps others to cross.

GLOSSARY

GLOSSARY

ahamkāra   I-consciousness.

ahimsā   Non-injury.

ākāśa   The first of the five material elements that constitute the universe; often translated as "space" and "ether." The four other elements are vāyu (air), agni (fire), ap (water), and prithivi (earth).

animā   Minuteness; one of the supernatural powers, by which a yogi can make himself as small as an atom.

antahkarana   The inner organ; the mind.

apāna   That modification of the vital breath in the body by which unassimilated food and drink are eliminated. See prāna.

āpta   An illumined person, whose words are infallible.

āptavākya   The words of an illumined person.

āsana   Posture.

Ātman   The Self or Soul; denotes both the Supreme Soul and the individual soul.

Bhagavad Gitā   An important Hindu scripture, comprising eighteen chapters of the epic *Mahābhārata* and containing the teachings of Śri Krishna.

bhakta   Devotee of God.

Bharata   A king who in old age retired to the forest to lead a holy life. According to the legend, he cherished at the time of death the thought of his pet deer and therefore was reincarnated as a deer.

Brahman   The Absolute; the Supreme Reality of the Vedānta philosophy.

Brahma Sutras   An authoritative treatise on the Vedānta philosophy, ascribed to Vyāsa.

287

brāhmin   A member of the priestly caste, the highest caste in Hindu society.

buddhi   The determinative faculty of the mind, which makes decisions; sometimes translated as "intellect."

chitta   The mind-stuff; that part of the inner organ which is the storehouse of memory or which seeks for pleasurable objects.

devas   (Lit., shining ones.) The gods of Hindu mythology.

dhāranā   Fixing the mind on a point; a stage in the process of meditation.

dhyāna   Concentration.

eight powers   The supernatural powers manifested by the yogi, such as the ability to make himself subtle as an atom, light as cotton, all-pervasive, etc.

Ganapati   Also known as Ganeśa, the Hindu deity with an elephant's head.

Gārgi   A woman seer mentioned in the Vedas.

Gāyatri   A sacred verse of the Vedas recited daily by Hindus of the three upper castes after their investiture with the sacred thread.

Gitā   Same as Bhagavad Gitā.

gunas   A term of the Sāmkhya philosophy, according to which prakriti (nature or matter), in contrast with Purusha (Soul), consists of three gunas—usually translated as "qualities"—known as sattva, rajas, and tamas. Tamas stands for inertia, rajas for activity or restlessness, and sattva for balance or wisdom.

guru   Spiritual preceptor.

hatha-yoga   A school of yoga that aims chiefly at physical health and well-being.

hatha-yogi   One who practises the disciplines of hatha-yoga.

Hum   A mystic word mentioned in the Tantra philosophy.

Iḍā   A nerve in the spinal column. See Sushumnā.

Indra   The king of the gods.

indriyas   The sense-organs, consisting of the five organs of perception, the five organs of action, and the mind.

Iśvara   The Personal God.

kaivalya   The term used in Rāja-yoga for ultimate liberation, meaning independence of the soul from the body or matter.

Kapila   The founder of the Sāmkhya philosophy.

karma   Action in general; duty. The Vedas use the word chiefly to denote ritualistic worship and humanitarian action.

Krishna   An Incarnation of God described in the *Mahābhārata* and the *Bhāgavata Purāna*.

kumbhaka   Retention of the breath; a process in prānāyāma, or breath-control, described in rāja-yoga and hatha-yoga.

Kundalini   (Lit., coiled-up serpent.) The word refers to the spiritual power dormant in all living beings. When awakened through the practice of spiritual disciplines, it rises through the spinal column, passes through various centres, and at last reaches the brain, whereupon the yogi experiences samādhi, or total absorption in the Godhead. See Sushumnā.

lotus   Each of the six centres along the Sushumnā is called a lotus, since their form is like that of a lotus blossom. See Kundalini.

Mādhyamikas   A school of Buddhist philosophers.

Mahābhārata   A celebrated Hindu epic.

mahat   The cosmic mind

manas   The faculty of doubt and volition; sometimes translated as "mind."

mantra   Sacred word by which a spiritual teacher initiates his disciple; Vedic hymn; sacred word in general.

Nāda   The mystic word *Om,* the symbol of Brahman.

nāḍi   Nerve.

Nārada   A saint in Hindu mythology.

niyama   Restraint of the mind; the second of the eight Yoga disciplines.

Nyāya   Indian logic; founded by Gautama, it is one of the six systems of orthodox Hindu philosophy.

ojas   Virility.

Om   The most sacred word of the Vedas; also written Aum. It is a symbol both of the Personal God and of the Absolute.

Patanjali   The author of the Yoga system, one of the six systems of orthodox Hindu philosophy, which deals with concentration and its methods, control of the mind, and similar matters.

Pingalā   A nerve in the spinal column. See Sushumnā.

prakriti   Primordial nature; the material substratum of the creation, consisting of sattva, rajas, and tamas.

prāna   The vital breath, which sustains life in a physical body; the primal energy or force, of which other physical forces are manifestations. In the books of Yoga, prāna is described as having five modifications, according to its five bodily functions: (1) prāna (which controls the breath), (2) apāna (which carries downward unassimilated food and drink), (3) vyāna (which pervades the entire body), (4) udāna (by which the contents of the stomach are ejected through the mouth, and by which the soul is conducted from the body at death), and (5) samāna (which carries nutrition throughout the body).

prānāyāma   Control of the breath; one of the disciplines of Yoga.

pratyāhāra   Restraining the organs.

Purānas   Books of Hindu mythology.

Purusha   (Lit., person.) A term of the Sāmkhya philosophy denoting the individual conscious principle. In Vedānta the term *Purusha* denotes the Self.

rajas   The principle of restlessness or activity in nature. See gunas.

Rāja-yoga   A system of yoga ascribed to Patanjali, dealing with concentration and its methods, control of the mind, samādhi, and similar matters.

rāja-yogi   One who follows the disciplines of Rāja-yoga.

Ramakrishna   A great saint of Bengal (A.D. 1836-1886), regarded as a Divine Incarnation.

rechaka   The rejecting or exhaling of the breath.

Rig-Veda   One of the four Vedas. See Vedas.

samādhi   Ecstasy, trance, communion with God.

Samhitā   A section of the Vedas containing a collection of hymns.

Sāmkhya   Founded by Kapila, it is one of the six systems of orthodox Hindu philosophy; it teaches that the universe evolves as the result of the union of prakriti (nature) and Purusha (Spirit).

samskāra   Mental impression or tendency created by an action.

samyama   A spiritual discipline in Rāja-yoga which combines concentration (dhāranā), meditation (dhyāna), and total absorption (samādhi).

Sankara   Same as Sankarāchārya.

Śankarāchārya   One of the greatest saints and philosophers of India (A.D. 788-820), the foremost exponent of Non-dualistic Vedānta.

sattva   The principle of balance or righteousness in nature. See gunas.

sāttvikas   Those in whom the quality of sattva is greatly developed.

Self   The same as Brahman, or Pure Spirit.

self   The individual self.

siddhis   The supernatural powers possessed by a yogi, such as the ability to make himself subtle as an atom, light as cotton, all-pervasive, etc.

soma   A creeper whose juice was used in Vedic sacrifices.

Soul   The same as Brahman, or Pure Spirit.

soul   The individual soul.

Śri   The word is often used as an honorific prefix to the names of deities and eminent persons, or of celebrated books generally of a sacred character.

Sushumnā   The Sushumnā, Idā, and Pingalā are the three most prominent nāḍis, or nerves, among the innumerable nerves in the nervous system. Of these, again, the Sushumnā is the most important, lying between the other two and being their point of harmony. The Idā is on the left side, and the Pingalā on the right. The Sushumnā, through which the awakened spiritual energy rises, is described as the Brahmavartman, or Pathway to Brahman. It is situated within the spinal column and extends from the base of the spine to the brain. See Kundalini.

sutra   Aphorism.

Svāti   The star Arcturus, regarded as forming the fifteenth lunar asterism.

Śvetāśvatara Upanishad   One of the major Upanishads. See Upanishads.

Swami   (Lit., lord.) A title of the monks belonging to the Vedānta school.

tamas   The principle of dullness or inertia in nature. See gunas.

tanmātras   The subtle elements of matter as originally evolved.

Tantra   A system of religious philosophy in which the Divine Mother, or Power, is regarded as Ultimate Reality; also the scriptures dealing with this philosophy.

udāna   That modification of the vital breath in the body by which the contents of the stomach are ejected through the mouth and by which the soul is conducted from the body at death. See prāna.

Upanishads   The well-known Hindu scriptures containing the philosophy of the Vedas. They are one hundred and eight in number, of which eleven are called major Upanishads.

vairāgya   Renunciation.

Vāmadeva   A sage in Hindu mythology.

Vedānta   (Lit., the essence or concluding part of the Vedas.) A system of philosophy mainly based upon the teachings of the Upanishads, the Bhagavad Gitā, and the *Brahma Sutras*.

Vedas   The revealed scriptures of the Hindus, consisting of the Rig-Veda, Sāma-Veda, Yajur-Veda, and Atharva-Veda.

Vivasvān   The sun god.

viveka   Discrimination between the real and the unreal.

vritti   State; form.

Vyāsa   The compiler of the Vedas, reputed author of the *Mahābhārata* and the *Brahma Sutras,* and father of the sage Śukadeva.

Vyāsa Sutras   Same as *Brahma Sutras.*

Yājnavalkya   A sage described in the *Brihadāranyaka Upanishad* as a knower of Brahman.

yama   Self-restraint, the first of the eight steps of Rāja-yoga.

yoga   Union of the individual soul and the Supreme Soul. The discipline by which such union is effected. The yoga system of philosophy, ascribed to Patanjali, is one of the six systems of orthodox Hindu philosophy; it deals with the realization of Truth through the control of the mind.

yogi   One who practises yoga.

Yudhishthira   One of the heroes of the *Mahābhārata;* the eldest of the five sons of Pāndu.

INDEX

INDEX

Absolute: and manifestation, 94 ff.
ākāśa, 34
āsana, 22, 23, 89, 178-79, 225, 232

chitta, 102 ff.; manifestations of, 104-05. *See also* mind
Christ, 282
concentration, 13-14; on different objects, 132-34. *See also* meditation, samādhi, superconsciousness

desire, 212
dhāranā, 22, 70, 90, 132-34, 181, 183
dhyāna, 22, 83, 90, 183. *See also* meditation, concentration, samādhi, superconsciousness
discipleship, 270 ff.; preparations for, 271 ff.

egoity, 147
endurance, 275
ethics, 78
evolution, 206-08

food, 20-1
freedom: desire for, 283 ff.

God, 118
gods, 119 ff.
gunas, 160 ff.
guru, 277 ff.

hatha-yoga, 23-4
heaven, 271-72

Idā, *see* Sushumnā
ignorance, 146, 168
instinct, 37-8, 149

kaivalya, 200, 203, 220
karma, 157, 191
Knowledge: steps to, 170-72
kriyā-yoga, 143 ff.
Kundalini, 50 ff., 57
Kurma Purāna, 87

meditation, 84-5; object of, 91; result of, 135. *See also* concentration, dhyāna, samādhi, superconsciousness
mind, 15, 19, 102 ff.; modifications of, 105 ff.; control of, 110; 214 ff.;